ENHANCING YOUR LIFE NOW

Four Basic Principles to Achieving Wellness

AVIVA PUBLISHING
New York

Dr. Jeudi Boulom, DC

Enhancing Your Life Now

How to Create Your Wellness with Four Basic Principals

Address all inquiries to:

Dr. Jeudi Boulom, DC

www.EnhancingYourLifeNow.com

ISBN: 978-1-935586-13-5

Library of Congress Control Number: 2010908436

Editor: Tyler R. Tichelaar, Ph.D.

Cover Design/Interior Layout: Fusion Creative Works, www.fusioncw.com

Printed in the United States of America

For additional copies, visit: www.EnhancingYourLifeNow.com

DEDICATION

To my beautiful children, Faith and Thomas Boulom: Thank you for your understanding that Mommy sometimes has to take time off from play to work on this book. You both are the reasons that inspired me to continue searching for a better solution to health. I hope as you become adults, you will become experts on health and take care of your bodies with great love and respect.

To Sky: Thank you for your patience and understanding. Thank you for making sure our children are the key factor behind every decision we make.

To my dear father, Soeung K. Taing: Thank you for your wisdom and for your desire to give all your children a better life in America. You are not only loved by your children, but by all who are fortunate enough to know you.

To all my siblings, Olivia, Dean, Lin, Hong, Putbory, Mardi, Mercredi, and Sam: you are the greatest siblings I could ever have. I love you all. It's such a joy to see you all successful in life.

To you, the reader: It is a joy and honor to help you have better knowledge about your body so you can create and achieve optimal health.

ACKNOWLEDGEMENTS

This book is the absolute result of all the great masterminds who have come before me to lay the groundwork for those of us who desire to seek more knowledge and understanding of how intricate our lives are with Mother Nature and our surrounding environment. It is such a great pleasure to have known or to have studied the works of some of the great healers of Alternative Care such as: Dr. Royal Lee, DDS; Dr. Weston Price, DDS; Dr. Harvey W. Wiley, MD, PhD; Dr. John H. Tilden, MD; Dr. Ronald Schmidt, ND; Dr. Lawrence Wilson, MD; Dr. Paul C. Eck; Dr. D.D. Palmer, DC; Dr. BJ Palmer, DC; Dr. James W. Parker, DC; Dr. Chester A. Wilk, DC; Dr. Terry A. Rondberg, DC; Dr. John Brimhall, DC; Dr. Craig Ross, DC; Dr. Joel Alcantera, DC; and Dr. Eric Berg. I have learned so much from these great mastermind teachers and healers, and I am so grateful to have had the opportunity to meet some of them.

This book would not be possible without the behind the scenes work of my great editor Tyler Tichelaar, for his grace, skilled knowledge, and kind communication style, or without the help of my wonderful agent, Patrick Snow, for his great coaching skill and continued support.

And of course to all my dear patients over the years who have put their health and trust in me. Thank you so much for believing in me and for your honest testimonials.

Last but not least, thank you to all my dear friends and family for your support and your belief in me.

CONTENTS

INTRODUCTION

I was inspired to write this book because we live in a country full of abundance, yet millions of Americans are living without health insurance and over a hundred thousand Americans are dying every year due to medical errors that could have been avoided. According to the World Health Organization (WHO), the United States spends a higher portion of its Gross Domestic Product (GDS) on healthcare than any other nation, yet it ranks 37 out of 191 countries in terms of the basic health of its citizens. Healthcare costs in the United States have become unaffordable for the average working family, and given the economic hardships of recent years, including job layoffs, health insurance has become even more difficult to afford. Millions of Americans have even decided to drop their health insurance because of its cost despite the dire consequences if they ever get sick. Furthermore, according to the *American Journal of Medicine*, more than 60 percent of bankruptcies filed by Americans are due to medical bills, and that number increased by 50 percent from 2001 to 2007. Believe it or not, middle class, well-educated families filed most of those bankruptcy claims. Plus, more than 75 percent of the medical-billed bankruptcies filed were from people who had insurance, yet the insurance was not enough to cover their bills, even though insurance premiums continue to rise at an astounding rate.

Obviously, the problems of healthcare are serious and costly. In the U.S. alone, $400 billion a year is spent just to treat heart disease and $200 billion a year to treat cancer. Thus, health has become a commodity, and it is a very expensive commodity. Those who are healthy are very blessed.

Although President Barack Obama and Congress worked very hard to finalize the healthcare bill that will help to sustain the rising costs of healthcare, we as American citizens can assist in resolving this enormous crisis. We have the responsibility to work with the government and our communities to correct this devastating crisis that has bankrupted many American families and our economy. This crisis requires each and every one of us to take action in order to rein in the cost and prevent more lives from being lost to unnecessary medical procedures and unnecessary medications. We can begin by applying today the principle steps to investing in our health to create a better future for our children and our own health. I will present those investment principles in this book.

Ask not what your country can do for you; ask what you can do for your country.
— President John F. Kennedy

In this book, I have incorporated information that will hopefully stimulate you into taking action to create a healthy lifestyle for your family and for yourself. I have organized the book around four basic investment principles that are the foundation and key to achieving optimal health. Once you understand the reasons behind these principles and begin to apply them to your life, achieving optimal health and saving money will be the return on your investment. Investing in our health is just like anything else in life; it requires an understanding of the basic principles required to achieve our goal. And I believe American citizens want to be healthy and do what is right for themselves and their families; they are just confused about how to make that investment. This book will answer how.

For instance, we all know that investing for our retirement requires that we understand the fundamental rules of investing and that we also have money to invest. And there are numerous resources about how to save money and invest for retirement. However, few books have focused on investing to create a healthy life. And yet, 60 percent of all bankruptcies in the U.S. are the result of medical expenses for the treatment of chronic ailments. Now, why is that? Here we are living in the richest country in the world, we have the most advanced technologies in the world, and we have many of the smartest people in the world, yet we are one of the world's sickest nations—ranked 37 out of 191. Plus, according to a 2007 survey, healthcare spending grew 6.1 percent while our GDP grew 2 percent in the U.S. Over 40 million Americans are without insurance, and hundreds of thousands of deaths annually result from medical negligence. Also, the costs of healthcare continue to rise each year. These statistics are so alarming. No wonder most Americans have started to look for alternative ways to address their health and their illnesses.

America's healthcare system is neither healthy, caring, nor a system.

—Walter Cronkite

Therefore, investing and creating healthy living should be the first priority especially when 60 percent of all bankruptcies are the result of medical expenses. If we want to retire and enjoy all of our life's savings, we must understand why we need to invest in our health now and not later. And the focus should be an emphasis on how to invest properly into our health so it will not cost us an arm and a leg now or a lifetime to fix the problems later. So creating healthy living is just like any goal or dream we have set for ourselves. For instance, have you ever dreamt of becoming a great singer, football player, doctor, lawyer, or writer? Whatever the vision you hold for yourself, when you have a goal you want to achieve, you have to follow through with a well-thought-out plan. Understanding basic principles and following steps to achieve those principles is required to enjoy optimal health.

So investing for retirement should be secondary to investing in healthy living because without our health, no amount of money is going to save our lives. And besides, a serious ailment may require our entire savings plus more with no guarantee we will be healed. Thus, when we choose to create healthy lifestyles in our homes and families by adopting the four basic investment principles of healthy living, everyone we love will experience a healthier future.

And the greatest news is that we are the ones who hold the answers and the key to our health, life, and future. No one else has more control and more say in what we do, how we feel, and what happens to us than our very own selves! So why not spend some time and money investing in our health today? Start with small steps to create a healthy life for your family and yourself by spending a little more money now. Buy organic foods that are healthy for your body; spend money on things like chemical free products that support your overall health; invest some time in proper exercise, detoxify your body from all the toxins, and get regular spinal care. Don't wait until your body gives up and it becomes expensive to treat the conditions.

Once you fall off the cliff, it is too late to get help;
therefore, get help before you fall off the cliff.
— Chinese Proverb

Thus, to create an optimal wellness for our families and ourselves, we must apply the four basic principles of wellness that I will cover throughout the rest of this book.

The Four Basic Principles of Wellness:

1. Good Nutrition

2. Daily Exercise

3. Removal of Toxins

4. Regular Spinal Care

Healthy citizens are the greatest asset any country can have.

— Winston Churchill

Section 1

NUTRITION

Let food be thy medicine and medicine thy food.
– Hippocrates

Chapter 1

THE NEED FOR HEALTHY EATING

Although there is a great deal of controversy among scientists about the effects of ingested food on the brain, no one denies that you can change your cognition and mood by what you eat.

– Arthur Winter

Living in America is like living in Heaven. We have abundance surrounding us daily in the form of food, shelter, and technology. And the greatest thing about living in America is that we have choices. We have a choice in every aspect of our lives. We can choose to be rich, poor, happy, sad, angry, strong, weak, sick, or healthy. Yes, health is also a choice. All these choices are there for us to choose from unlike in other countries where your right to choose is limited.

When I was a little girl growing up in Cambodia, not only was our right to freedom taken from us, but so was our right to food, shelter, to be with our families, and to have control over our health. During the Khmer Rouge government, the nation's leaders not only stripped away our freedom to live in our own homes with our families, but they limited our contact with our loved ones, our sleep, our water, and our food. My sister and I were separated from our aunts and placed in an all girl camp where the girls were all about five or six years old. I believe I was the youngest in the group. Our job was to act as scarecrows in the rice fields, to pick up cow dung for fertilizer, and to chop up some leaves to mix with cow manure to make fertilizer for the rice. Food was very scarce. All the children worked the entire day long without water or food. Our only meal was at dinnertime and that was rice mixed with sweet potatoes.

Thus, when I first arrived in America, I could not believe my eyes when I went shopping with my family at the Safeway supermarket. There was a vast abundance of everything from fruits and vegetables to all kind of meats. I felt like I had died and gone to Heaven. Anyone would experience this feeling who came to America from a war-torn country where throughout your childhood all you had to eat were crickets, grasshoppers, and plants. Seeing such an abundance of food in America was beyond belief to me!

The first time I ever tasted real chicken meat was in 1979. That was the year when Vietnamese soldiers came into Cambodia to fight the Khmer Rouge. All the Cambodian citizens ran and hid in different places away from the Khmer Rouge. My sister and I managed to locate our aunts in the midst of all the gunshots and people running everywhere; we left where we were and settled in a new village. Soon after, I had a three-day fever and was unconscious most of the time. My aunt went out and caught a chicken and prepared it for our family. Oh how sweet, juicy, and delicious that chicken tasted! That was the best experience of my life. I completely regained my energy after eating that chicken. So to walk into a place where every kind of food imaginable was within reach just put me in awe.

American citizens are the luckiest people in the world. They live a heavenly life filled with bountiful food, shelter, and the freedom to choose how they want to live. However, with all that abundance comes a price if we are not careful; while food may be bountiful, not all of that food is healthy for our bodies.

Therefore, knowing what is good for our body, and whether or not we choose to practice healthy eating depends on what we want for the future outcome of our health. How healthy do you want to be? What is the condition of health you want to have, and what kind of health will you have if you continue to eat the way you are currently eating? What we eat today will determine our overall health tomorrow. Thus, when we choose to eat healthy foods in moderation, our body will use up the food's nutrients and convert them into energy or build stronger bodies for us from those nutrients. But if we eat unhealthy foods, then the body has no nutrients to build on so the brain sends out a signal to increase hunger, which makes us want to eat more. It's this hunger that triggers our overeating, which in turn leads to our being overweight and undernourished in America. In other words, our Standard American Diet (SAD) is creating our health crisis!

Undernourishment is defined as suffering from lack of food or nourishment. Americans are certainly not lacking in food—in fact, we like to super size our meals. So our undernourishment is the result of our not eating the right kinds of food that will nourish our bodies.

Our concept of eating needs to be adjusted from "Eat for pure enjoyment" to "Eat to nourish your body." I know a lot of people feel they should be able to enjoy the food they eat because they deserve it. But, if our body had a say in it, it would reply, "I deserve to be fed healthy, nourishing food, so I can use those vitamins and minerals to keep you alive!"

I remember my dad used to say that if he couldn't enjoy the foods he loved to eat, there was no point in living. However, he changed his thinking when he started to develop gout in his big toe every time he ate something he shouldn't; he now has a better understanding and appreciation of how certain foods affect his overall health. Gout is an acute recurrent inflammation that usually is hot, red, tender, and causes swelling of the joints. Having gout can change a person's eating habits immediately. And only those living with gout understand the excruciating pain.

The correlation between our health and what we eat has been understood since the time of Hippocrates, the father of modern medicine, in the fourth century B.C. It was Hippocrates who said, "Let food be thy medicine and medicine be thy food." He truly meant that food is our most effective (miracle) medicine on the planet. No medicine is more healing than the nourishment found in food. Nourishing food is a medicine without side-effects, and it is very cheap compared to prescription medication. For instance, beets are a very good source of vitamin A, C, biotin, and niacin. They are also rich in phosphorous, sodium, magnesium, calcium, iron, potassium, folic acid, and fiber. The ancient Greeks used beets for blood cooling, and the Roman used beets to fight fever. Recent research shows that eating beet juices slows down the development of tumors. Furthermore, Dr. **H.C.A. Vogel, in** *The Nature Doctor*, **states that the betaine found in beet juice is known to stimulate the functions of liver cells and protect the liver and bile ducts; thus, patients with liver conditions can greatly benefit from this amazing vegetable.**

Remember how Popeye the Sailor was always getting beat up by Bluto until he ate his can of spinach? Once Popeye had his spinach, he suddenly had the energy and strength to fight Bluto and win. Did you ever wonder why the creators of that cartoon chose spinach? It's because spinach is a rich source of antioxidants, of vitamins A, C, E, K, and of folic acid, magnesium, iron, calcium, potassium, zinc, copper, selenium, phosphorus, protein, niacin, and omega-3 fatty acids. Spinach is one of the most nutrient rich vegetables. It contains over twenty different vitamins and minerals.

How about kale? It's a green leafy vegetable that is so rich in calcium, lutein, iron, and vitamins A, C, and K. Plus, kale contains a naturally rich sulfur content called sulforaphane, which helps the liver to detoxify cancer-causing chemicals found in items to which we are daily exposed. Furthermore, sulforaphane is known to help stop breast cancer cell proliferation as reported by the *Journal of Nutrition* (2004). So if you are looking in the store for vitamins or minerals that contain all the ingredients our body needs and that have a very powerful healing effect, then look no further. Eating these foods on a daily basis not only supplies the body with the right amount of vitamins and minerals, but the nutrients from them will actually prevent the possibility of having cancer, arthritis, constipation, and many other ailments.

The need for healthy eating really comes down to giving our body the raw material it needs to build strong cells as a foundation for our future health. And by supplying the nutrients to our body, we decrease our appetite for more junk food because the brain is now satisfied with the nutrients it received from raw vegetables and fruits. Furthermore, with all the stress that bombards us, it is essential that we provide our bodies with some support by taking small steps like healthy eating. However, if we don't eat the right types of food, thus depriving our body of the nutrients it needs, we will have cravings for certain foods so our body can acquire the minerals and vitamins needed to meet its demand. For instance, when you crave chocolate, chances are your body is deficient in magnesium and chocolate contains magnesium. And if you crave something sweet, it could be that your body is deficient in potassium. Potassium is required to convert all the excess sugar that we eat into glycogen. Glycogen is a reserve form of energy that can easily be accessed to meet the body's energy demands.

Eating properly really isn't that difficult. Yet Americans seem to be confused by the mixed messages from the media and the health experts about what to eat and what not to eat. For example, should we eat carbohydrates or not? How about whether we should avoid salt? Should we eat fat or no fat? Should we become vegetarians or is eating meat actually better for us?

In actuality, our body needs everything, but in moderation. Our body needs carbohydrates so it can break them down into sugar to use as energy. And our body needs salts for the nerve and muscle functions and to absorb major nutrients and maintain an adequate balance of water and minerals. We need proteins to build muscles and everything else that keeps our body healthy and strong. Plus, our body needs fats to give the cell membranes permeability, to produce hormones, and to absorb fat soluble vitamins like A, E, and K. We need fruits and vegetables for the vitamins and minerals found in them. So carbohydrates, meat, and salt are not what are making us unhealthy; instead it's the type of carbohydrates, salts, and meats we are consuming.

To understand how our body uses the vitamins and minerals we consume to build strong cells, picture a carpenter building a house. The carpenter uses such raw materials as lumber, sheetrock, nails, etc. to build a new home. He must choose different materials to construct a custom built home compared to the materials he would use to build just another mass-produced home. Since a custom built home is more expensive, the builder needs to be more detailed and requires higher quality raw materials. The same situation applies to the body. When we choose whether to eat junk food or nourishing food, our body will tell us almost immediately whether that food was high quality or low quality by how we feel after—do we have more energy, or are we tired, sleepy, or running to the bathroom within a couple of hours after we eat? To continue with our home-building analogy, let's look at the Three Little Pigs.

Remember the story of the Three Little Pigs? Remember who built the strongest house? Would you rather live in the straw, stick, or brick home? Let's look at three groups of people whom we can compare with the Three Little Pigs.

GROUP 1: THE HOUSE BUILT OF STRAW

In the story, the first pig went out and gathered up some straw and built his home rather quickly. He did not know that Mr. Wolf had very strong lungs and could easily blow his house down. Had the first little pig just taken the time to understand why it is important from the beginning to build a strong home with a good foundation, even though it takes a little bit longer to complete, he would have been safe from the wolf.

The first little pig did what was quick and easy. Similarly when it comes to eating, many people will choose whatever foods are fast and convenient for them and their families. They do not have time to cook a hot meal, they don't read labels, and they may not be concerned with where the foods originated. They might lack the information needed to make good food choices, or they might simply be lazy. For example, one of my siblings would rather eat what is convenient and readily available to her than to make the effort to prepare healthy food for her body. She also loves to wait until her body starves, which makes her very hungry, so she needs something quick to satisfy her hunger. This practice is bad because when you are hungry, you tend to eat unhealthy food which just makes your body feel worse. The fast or convenient food may satisfy your hunger temporarily, but if the food has no nutritious value, it just makes the body work harder to process it, using up more energy to rid your body of the toxins you just put inside.

For children especially, this situation can be detrimental. Fast and convenient foods for children such as fried chicken, French fries, JoJO's, candy, crackers, refined cakes, and soft drinks make up the Standard American Diet (SAD). On this diet, a child's dietary intake of omega-6 to omega-3 is anywhere from 10:1 to 30:1. The lower the ratio the better, and most doctors and nutritionists recommend a ratio below 4:1. But this fast food diet's large amount of omega-6 triggers a weak intestinal wall, which leads to chronic inflammation and ultimately to such diseases as asthma, diabetes, and obesity. Plus, this food does not have enough nutrients to allow children's bodies to build new cells. Obesity then results because their little bodies need more nutrients, so their brains trigger the hunger mechanism to continue eating more and more, until the proper nutrients are supplied to the body; that is why they overeat—their bodies are crying out for nourishment to build strong bones, form red blood cells, strengthen hormones, and metabolize fats, protein, and carbohydrates. However, because the diets are deficient in nutrients, the body starts to break down faster than it is able to rebuild new cells.

When I am eating more organic greens with some organic coconut oil in my meal, I feel very stable and satisfied throughout the day, but when I eat only refined foods such as a chicken burger and French fries, I find myself feeling hungry all the time, so I need to eat something more. The reason is that my body cannot find many useful nutrients in refined carbohydrate foods like a hamburger and fries compared to a plate of salad with avocado, coconut oil, and some almond nuts tossed on top.

Furthermore, by the time children have grown older, their taste buds have acquired the taste of all those refined foods and additives so they find eating fresh fruits and vegetables to be very bland. For example, one of my patients always complains about how her children will not drink water and will not eat soups, but when she buys a case of soda, it is gone within two days. Most Americans prefer drinking soda over water or eating pizza over nourishing vegetable dips. This preference has become the norm of almost every household in America, and parents have given into it because they worry that if they don't buy or prepare the food their children love to eat, their children will not eat and instead starve. Most parents fail to realize that by giving into their children's demands, they are not nourishing their children but actually doing more harm to their health.

So children continue to eat fast foods, refined carbohydrates, refined sugars, and drink more soda and coffee. And they sit while they play video games or watch television, which leads to health problems like diabetes, hypertension, and obesity. These diseases are the direct result of over-consumed refined carbohydrates that stimulate insulin release, which then causes the body to store these excess refined carbohydrates as fats and cholesterol instead of using them for energy. This lifestyle is what has put our children's health at risk and caused them to acquire diseases previously only found in adults.

According to Dr. Baillie-Hamilton, the author of *Stop the 21st Century Killing You*, "if the nutritional deficiency continues for any length of time, this too tends to lead to an increased risk of developing one of the many auto-immune diseases." Furthermore, a recent report in the *New England Journal of Medicine* warned that unless obesity in Americans is reduced, today's youth will live less healthy and possibly shorter lives than their parents because every day, due to a nutrient deficiency, they are breaking down cells faster than they are building new ones.

Worthless people live only to eat and drink;
people of worth eat and drink only to live.
— Socrates

As parents, we cannot continue to feed our children refined carbohydrates, refined sugars, and artificial flavors and colors. Our children's bodies need all the essential nutrients to build strong, vibrant cells and healthy immune functions so they can combat all the constant stresses that our children are facing on a daily basis.

Tell me what you eat, and I will tell you what you are.
— Anthelme Brillat-Savarin

GROUP 2: THE HOUSE BUILT OF STICKS

As for the second little piggy who built his house out of sticks, in his mind, he was building a strong home. But we all know what happened to the little piggy and his home.

In this second group, the individuals are doing their best to feed their families well. They buy fresh vegetables, they cook homemade meals, and they drink plenty of water to nourish their bodies. However, they are still getting sick because of such factors as a depletion of nutrients in the soil, the way they prepare their meals, the type of salt and sugar they use, and unhealthy oil they use for cooking. For instance, since vegetables are sensitive to heat, cooking them in high heat as in a stir fry or boiling them in a soup will destroy the essential nutrients in them that your body needs. Our body receives the highest level of nutrients from vegetables when they are eaten raw in their natural form. And because our soil has fewer nutrients in it today than it had a century ago, we need to eat more fruits and vegetables then ever before.

Cooking oil has caused a lot of confusion because different oils are better for different menus; the best oil to use when cooking with high heat is coconut oil because it is very stable compared to vegetable oils like canola or corn oil. Corn oil has a very high ratio of omega-6 to omega-3 (46:1). The best oil for salads or low heat cooking is olive oil. The best additional supplement would be flax seed oil or fish oil.

Another confusing topic is salt. Sea salt is the answer to the quandary of whether to eat salt or not have salt. We need to remember that are body is largely composed of salt (sodium). Our body needs sodium for many functions including moving our muscles, balancing our alkalinity/acidity levels, restoring good digestion, relieving allergies and skin diseases, and removing toxins from the body. The reason sea salt is better than table salt is how it is processed. Sea salt is created through the evaporation of sea water with very little processing, so the trace minerals and other elements are all intact, whereas because table salt is heavily processed, the necessary trace minerals and elements are destroyed and chemicals are added, including bleach and anti-caking agent.

Furthermore, the people in this second group are often sick because our foods are filled with such chemicals as hormones, additives, pesticides, and antibiotics, both in our meats and produce. Chemicals in our foods have a major impact on our overall health. Because they are toxic, they disrupt our endocrine system and upset our glands by producing hormones and competing for binding sites like hormone receptors; this situation causes havoc in the communication system between organs such as the thyroid or adrenal glands. Because our body communicates through the language of hormones, any false information leads to over-production or under-production of certain hormones, and ultimately, to such problems as thyroid conditions and Graves disease, which results from an over-activity of the thyroid glands or decreased metabolism function and weight gain from low thyroid hormones. Thus, chemicals like pesticides, herbicides, fungicides, and even prescription medications will all compete for the body's natural hormone production sites and thereby limit the body's ability for its different organs to communicate properly with each other. These toxic chemicals are found everywhere in our daily lives, but especially in our foods.

Some toxic chemicals found in our foods include:

Hormones: used in animal meats to make them gain weight which will reduce the feeding and waiting time before the slaughterhouse. In the dairy cow, hormones are used to increase the production of milk for more profit. Studies have shown that synthetic chemicals like hormones cause cancer. For instance, diethylstilbestrol (DES), a synthetic estrogen drug used in the 1960s, was withdrawn from use after it was found to increase the risk of vaginal cancer in daughters of treated women.

Food Additives: many are known to cause brain damage and water retention, which increases weight issues. Here is a breakdown of the problems caused by several and where they are typically found:

- **Acesulfame K** is used as a sweetener in gums, soda, and non-dairy creamers. It has been known to cause cancer in animals.

- **Aspartame** is included in such artificial sweeteners as Equal and NutraSweet. It is known to cause headaches, dizziness, epileptic-like seizures, and menstrual problems.
- **MSG** is found in Chinese foods, chips, and chicken broths. It is known to cause headaches, burning sensations in the forearm, and to damage brain cells. It also causes the body to retain water.
- **Nitrite** is found in several foods including lunchmeats, sausage, hot dogs, and crackers. It has been known to cause cancer.

Antibiotics are familiar to all of us and we know what they do—kill harmful bacteria. Why are antibiotics used in our foods, especially in such meats as poultry, beef, and pork? The main reason is to prevent animals from contracting infections, which will hurt the farmer's bottom line. Over two hundred tons of antibiotics are used for growth promotion in livestock. Whatever the animal eats stays in its system, and by extension, it is passed into our bodies when we consume animal products.

Pesticides: used to prevent bugs and insects from eating farmers' crops. The fruits and vegetables in our supermarkets today all contain residue from pesticides. Pesticides are known to be carcinogenic and to disrupt the endocrine system. According to the World Resources Institute, pesticides are the likely cause of immune suppression for millions of people throughout the world.

Other additional factors besides food affect our health including water, air, sleep, exercise, and poor intestinal absorption. Poor intestinal walls are the result of years of eating refined sugars, refined carbohydrates, taking medications, and consuming coffee and alcohol which overtime cause the intestinal walls to become weak and decrease their ability to absorb nutrients, thus decreasing the body's ability to be healthy. Because the absorption of all vitamins and minerals happens in the intestinal tracts of the small and large intestines, conditions such as constipation and irritable bowel syndrome ultimately limit the body's ability to absorb nutrients. However, if we continue to practice healthy eating, over time the damage done to our intestinal linings from poor eating and antibiotics will gradually heal and our intestines will be able to function fully again.

Furthermore, an unhealthy digestive tract limits our body's ability to care for itself, resulting in such health conditions as acne, constipation, low energy, and weight loss. Let's take a closer look at how unhealthy digestive walls cause these health conditions.

Intestinal Health and Constipation: The liver and kidneys are the major organs that filter out, detoxify, and eliminate the toxic chemicals in the body. When our intestinal lining is not working properly, our body is packed with waste and toxic substances that will cause the liver and kidneys to work extra hard to filter out the toxins. Constipation means that the waste in the intestinal walls causes our smooth muscle to be in a constant spastic mode which then limits the ability to absorb any nutrients. Smooth muscle contraction requires a lot of energy from the body to stay in contracting mode, which then takes energy away from the adrenal and thyroid glands, two of the body's major powerhouses for energy. If you are experiencing low energy, your body is busy taking care of its internal needs. Constipation, therefore, is worse than your just not being able to eliminate waste—it affects the health of your entire body.

Intestinal Health and Weight Loss: I see a lot of people who try to lose weight by trying all kind of products, only to end up being discouraged. I admit I have been one of those guilty people. If you are trying to lose weight by starving your body or by taking diet pills, you are looking at the wrong problem. These attempts to lose weight can be compared to someone who isn't a mechanic trying to find the plug to your car's red "service" light. Losing weight is difficult if you don't know what caused you to gain the weight in the first place. You may say, "I know what caused me to gain weight; it was because I ate a lot." But that is only a small part of how you gain weight. After all, why are some people able to eat large portions and eat frequently, yet they never gain weight?

My husband is such a person. I used to be jealous of him because he could eat anything and never gain a pound. By comparison, I would watch what I ate, sometimes skip dinner, and still have a hard time losing that extra twenty pounds I'd been trying to lose for the last ten years. What is the reason for the difference between my husband and me? It's because my body metabolizes very slowly compared to his and because my body is deficient in the vitamins and minerals needed to produce energy. Although, I believe I am healthy, my body tells me differently. I start to have constipation when I am overstressed by work, my children, or anything else I deal with daily. And constipation is a sign of slower metabolism, which results from my energy being drained by everything that causes me stress, and which in turn affects my thyroid and adrenal glands. According to scientist Paul Eck, the adrenal and thyroid glands are responsible for 98 percent of our body's energy production. And mine were constantly overworked not just from the external demands of my active everyday living, but also from having to produce the energy for my internal organs to do their work. As a result, I could not lose weight. I also have a poor tolerance for sugar because my body does not have enough energy or the minerals needed to convert sugar into energy. Plus, when I go to exercise, I just add more stress to my already stressed adrenal glands. So how can I lose weight? It's just not possible unless I correct the problem's source. The adrenal and the thyroid glands need to be at their optimal function, my intestinal walls need to be healthy, and my liver needs to be at its optimal level to filter out the toxins caused by the waste from constipation and all the other toxins that accumulate daily as I consume food. Once these issues are corrected, I have created a healthy environment for my body so that when I exercise, the weight will naturally come off without my having to try so hard.

Therefore, to understand why someone doesn't lose weight, it's important to look at the person's digestive tract and its functions. The majority of the time when someone has a weight problem, the digestive tract is very unhealthy.

Thus, losing weight by taking diet pills or skipping meals is a temporary solution, and it's the reason why people gain the weight back. Also, having a weak intestinal lining from an over-accumulation of toxins like yeast, candida, bacteria, and viruses can overcrowd our intestines and cause the intestinal linings to become weak and less permeable. Our liver is the major center for all fat burning hormone activities, so if the liver is weak due to an overload of toxins backed up in the intestinal lining, forcing the liver to detoxify all that recycled waste, it limits our body's ability to activate the liver to produce the fat burning hormones needed to burn the fat. Thus, if the nutrients that need to be absorbed into the bloodstream to build a strong body are limited, the body will trigger the hunger mechanism so the person will want to eat. The result is the cycle of obesity:

Body needs nutrients → Brain triggers hunger mechanism → We eat unhealthy foods → Body need nutrients → Brain triggers hunger mechanism → We continue to eat unhealthy foods → Unhealthy foods cause poor lining of the intestinal walls → Increased growth of yeast, bacteria, and viruses → Body is deficient in nutrients → We eat more unhealthy foods → Body stores unwanted fats and sugar as fats → Obesity

Intestinal Health and Beautiful Skin: Having a healthy intestinal lining helps the body to absorb the nutrients it needs to build stronger and more vibrant cells, which in turn makes your skin look radiant and beautiful. Furthermore, healthy intestinal walls prevent yeast, bacteria, and other food particles from entering the bloodstream, unlike when we have leaky gut syndrome where the intestinal walls are weak and allow the leakage of yeast, bacteria, and other particles into the bloodstream. Toxins that get deposited into the skin cause acne and other skin disorders.

I know from personal experience what it is to have acne. I had a severe outbreak of it when I was in high school. I tried everything from prescription ointment to cleaning my face four times a day. The more I cleaned my face, the more acne I had. It was huge acne with white heads. Even if I popped them, they would just keep on coming. It was a nightmare. The reason for my severe acne was that I would go all day without water, and I ate a lot of refined foods. I didn't realize that my face was paying the consequences of my failure to understand how food and water impact my health. I did not begin to understand the value of water and healthy eating until my first year of chiropractic school.

Intestinal Health and Energy: Most American tends to have low energy and to use coffee or energy drinks to give them a temporary boost. However, over time, these drinks take a toll on the adrenal glands and the thyroid. The adrenal glands and the thyroid are the power source for the body's energy production, so overstimulating them will eventually lead to their breakdown. Low energy, therefore, is a sign of a poor digestive tract from a poor eating lifestyle that has caused the adrenal glands and thyroid to work overtime until they burn out and malfunction. To have more energy, we must create healthy intestinal walls by choosing to eat greater quantities of healthy fruits and vegetables so we get higher levels of vitamins and minerals into the body, which the body will use to produce more energy and build stronger cells. For instance, the body needs calcium, magnesium, sodium, and potassium for the optimal functions of the thyroid and adrenal glands. The body requires the right balance of calcium to magnesium and sodium to potassium. According to scientist Paul Eck, the ideal ratio for calcium to magnesium should be 40/6 mg, and for sodium to potassium 25/10 mg. Anything less than these ratios will affect our energy level. Plus, these minerals are also needed in other parts of the body including the bones and nerve tissue, and they are necessary for enzyme production. The only way to acquire these minerals is to eat organic raw fruits and vegetables that are loaded with them. Raw fruits and vegetables contain a higher level of nutrients than when they are cooked. Similarly, natural vitamins and minerals come in small dosages with co-factors that help the body to absorb them, while synthetic vitamins only cause more harm to the body because they are not made from real live vegetables and fruits, but rather from coal tar and petroleum by-products.

Intestinal Health and Gray Hair: Did you know that gray hair is not the result of old age? My brother-in-law, who is the same age as me, has gray hair all over his head, but my aunt, who is twice my age, has barely any gray hair at all. Why is that?

Gray hair is our body's way of letting us know that our body is deficient in some vitamins and minerals due to a lack of nutrients in our diet and constant stress in our daily life. That stress is using up all of our body's energy, so we better do something quick or the fuel will soon run out. Gray hair is like a red light on the gas meter in our car, signaling us that we need to get more gas. We often hear people joke that their kids' behavior gives them gray hairs—this statement has some truth in it because stress can wreak havoc on the body. Stress is the consequence of failing to respond appropriately to emotional and physical threats, whether actual or imagined. Stress can be caused by such things as chronic pain, toxic food, the environment, and emotional situations such as divorce or financial problems. Not eating the proper foods can also create stress, which leads to gray hair.

For most people on the Standard American Diet, their daily food intake is loaded with refined carbohydrates and very few fruits and vegetables, so rather than nutrients, the body is being loaded down with an accumulation of free-radicals, and our weak intestinal linings, created by years of consuming refined carbohydrates in the form of cookies, candy, soda, and coffee, have limited our ability to absorb the nutrients. And then when we take antibiotics, we destroy the good bacteria in our intestinal walls that are not only necessary for our immune functions but vital for the production of vitamins B and K, and the absorption of other types of vitamins and minerals.

When the body doesn't have enough vitamins and minerals in its bloodstream, it has to steal from other places to create what is a first priority, such as our hormones, bones, and nerves. Thus, gray hair is a result of deficiency in manganese and iron. Manganese and iron are what make our hair color dark because the mineral colors are black. Also, manganese and iron are the two minerals the body needs to make energy. Plus, manganese is also used to help maintain healthy nerves, keep our thyroid functioning, make our bones strong, keep our blood sugar levels normal, and protect the cells from free-radicals. Therefore, our body steals from a place that has less priority, in this case our hair. So if we want to avoid getting gray hair, we must address the health of our digestive tract.

This second group of individuals, as I said earlier, may be eating healthier, but they may still not be consuming enough water, or the water they are consuming may be toxic to their bodies. The majority of Americans are chronically dehydrated. Dehydration is an excessive loss of body fluid. A great example of dehydration is grapes that have turned into raisins. Remember how plump and crunchy grapes are when you bite into them with their full water content? Consider the difference in texture to a raisin. The same thing happens to our body's internal organs when we don't drink enough water. Our skin and our organs shrink due to dehydration, which results in headaches, acne, asthma, and a host of other problems. On average, most Americans only consume two or three glasses of water per day; that even seems like a lot to some people. Because our body is composed of 70-80 percent water, we need water to cleanse our organs, to carry nutrients to the cells, to regulate body temperature, to drain toxins from the body, and for many other functions. When we exercise, we lose water through sweating. Bowel and urine elimination cause the body to lose water, and even exhaling when we breathe results in water loss. We lose on average six glasses of water per day, so drinking only two or three glasses of water daily is insufficient to replenish the body.

In addition, the caffeine in coffee and soda increases the body's water loss. The result of water loss is chronic dehydration, a major contributing factor to chronic inflammation, which in turn leads to numerous diseases including arthritis, asthma, skin disorder, constipation, hypertension, and cancer.

How about air? Obviously, we need the oxygen in air to survive. If we go without oxygen for more than a few minutes, we will die. That is how essential air is to the human body. Yet most Americans are shallow breathers, and sometimes, they are practically holding their breaths. Stop for a moment to observe yourself. Are you breathing so deeply that you see your belly rise and fall? That is how babies breathe and how we all should breathe. Few of us do, however, because we are so stressed with everything in our lives that we tend to hold in our breath. I am a shallow breather, and I catch myself holding my breath all the time. Not breathing deeply is bad because our bodies need air to convert into an energy called adenosine triphosphate (ATP). ATP is created inside mitochondria, which is known as the powerhouse of the cell. The amount of ATP produced depends on how much oxygen is available. ATP is used to help our heart pump blood to the rest of the body, and for our GI tract to grind food, absorb nutrients, and eliminate toxins from the body. As a result, a lack of ATP caused by shallow breathing leaves people more stressed and tired because the body cannot create the energy it needs to function properly.

GROUP 3: THE HOUSE BUILT OF BRICKS

Now, let's look at the third little piggy and how he handles his health. Obviously, the third little pig understood the importance of building a strong foundation, so he went out to find the strongest material to build his home—bricks. And we all know what happened to Mr. Wolf as a result, right?

The individuals in this third group take the time to research, read, and understand what they put into their food and their bodies. The majority of their diets consist of organic fruits and vegetables and organic meat. They usually eat raw nuts, raw vegetables in the form of juice or salads, and small portions of meat for protein. They also, exercise regularly to help the body remove any toxins that may have entered it unknowingly and to maintain their health. Often this third group has made this change because someone in the family had a condition that warranted healthy eating.

Do you remember Montel Williams, the talk show host who was diagnosed with Multiple Sclerosis (MS)? MS is a disease that affects the myelin sheath of the nerve, causing inflammation that results in the loss of the myelin sheath. Because of the pain and agony he experienced, Montel made a change to his diet and lifestyle. He sought out health professionals, including a nutritionist to teach him to eat properly and a chiropractor he visits regularly for chiropractic adjustments. Montel is now an expert on juicing and on healthy eating. He has inspired thousands of Americans to change the way they eat, and the result is that those people saw a dramatic drop in their weight.

How about Suzanne Somers? She is well known for her portrayal of a ditzy blonde on the television sitcom "Three's Company." A true fighter, when she was diagnosed with breast cancer that spread throughout her entire body, she changed her lifestyle. She studied nutrition, alternative forms of healthcare, and made the necessary changes. Today she is in complete remission and an active spokesperson for alternative treatments to cure cancer.

Lance Armstrong is another great story. He was diagnosed with testicular cancer that metastasized to his brain, abdomen, and lungs. His doctors gave him far less than a 50 percent survival chance. By choosing alternative forms of treatment, he not only beat his cancer, but he went on to win the Tour De France seven years in a row.

And what about Naomi Judd who was diagnosed with Hepatitis C? She was told she only had three years to live. But she changed her lifestyle and started to invest in her own health. Today, she is free and clear of Hepatitis C.

Jenny McCarthy's son is another example. He was diagnosed with autism after he received his vaccination shots. Her son is now cured from autism through lifestyle changes and diet. Jenny has gone on to become an advocate for parents of children with autism.

Finally, I am a member of this group of people who have overcome life-threatening illnesses for themselves or their children. I did not start to read, question, or research the importance of healthy eating or the value of food or water until December 27, 2000. On that day when we came back from the grocery store, I put my little boy, Thomas, to sleep on the bed and went back to get the groceries out of the car. I was just about to walk out the front door when a loud cry came from the bedroom. When I rushed to my son, I found him limp and with his eyes rolled back. There was no life force in him. I called the ambulance and took him to the children's hospital in Fort Worth where I spent the night with him. The ER doctors ran all the tests from a spinal tap to an MRI and an EKG. My son was diagnosed with febrile seizure. After that day, my little boy did not wake up; he just lay limp on the bed and sometimes would cry in the middle of the night. I sat and monitored his temperature every hour. Life became nothing more than Hell for me. I spent the next five years of his life basically trying to keep him from having seizures. We went the traditional route of medication and six month checkups with the doctor. But every month, we had to call an ambulance to transport us to the ER because he would go into a major convulsion. My adrenaline was always on the rise. I remember asking God why this situation had happened to me. I loved my son, and my husband and I were the best of parents to him so how could this be? How could parents who neglected their children end up with healthy sons and daughters while we loved our child so dearly only to have him suffer so much? The situation was not fair to him and not fair to us.

For the next four and a half years, I watched the doctors switch my little boy from one medicine to the next in an effort to try to help him, but every time the doctor switched his medicine or increased the dosage, Thomas would have more frequent seizures. Month after month, we ended up in the ER, and every time my son would be disturbed from his sleep due to routine hospital procedures to check his blood and temperature.

Our last visit to the ER was in 2004 when I nearly lost my little boy. He was not responding to any medication the ER doctors gave him. They had used up all their options. That day, he went into a seizure for more than four hours in the hospital ER. I thank the Lord for the ER doctor who was on staff that day. He gave us time to decide whether we wanted to go ahead and give Thomas more medicine. The risks involved were high. I remember just standing in the ER room crying my eyes out because I had no idea what to do. I prayed and prayed for help and for answers. Miraculously, thirty minutes later, my little boy came back. He was able to respond, which meant I no longer had to make a decision.

After that experience, I had reached the point where my maternal instinct kicked in. "Enough is enough," I told myself. "These doctors are more clueless than me when it comes to my little boy. They don't know him like I do since I am with him 24/7. They have no idea what this little boy is going through." I vowed then that I would do everything and anything to help Thomas be cured and to find the cure for this devastating condition.

I began seriously to look at Thomas' diet, at what triggered his seizures, and then to make some changes. It was a long journey to recovery, but by making changes to his diet, his seizures started to decrease drastically year after year. Before, he had been experiencing five to ten seizures a day, ranging from convulsions to Jacksonian, grand mal, and petite mal seizures that would knock him out and require him to sleep four to six hours afterwards. Today, he experiences at most just once a month an aura or salivation with minimal twitches. By correlation, his ability to understand and communicate took a leap forward each year. Today, Thomas eats more organic protein, less carbohydrates, and more organic fruits and vegetables. He has five small meals a day, and we walk twenty minutes each morning and afternoon, and if possible, also in the evening. He gets half of his body weight in fluids, and I make sure his surrounding environment is always calm and joyful. Everywhere we go, we pack homemade food made from fresh organic vegetables and organic meats. We eat fresh vegetable stir fry and soups with ingredients including sea salt and herbal plants, and everyday, I find new ways to improve our family's health.

So I am part of this third group of individuals, and like most of them, I changed my habits to include healthy eating because it was necessary. We individuals in this third group are overall very conscious of our health. We value health. To me, no price can be placed on being healthy because when you are sick, no amount of money can give you back the joy, time, and freedom to do what you want. Sickness limits your ability to experience and enjoy many things in life. For that reason, people in this group exercise regularly, eat a healthy breakfast, eat in moderation, and enjoy life. This group is at optimal health and willing to do whatever it takes to maintain it. Health is a privilege we don't want to lose.

Therefore, choosing healthy eating is the first key principle to investing in building a strong and healthy body. This investment costs just a small fraction of what you will pay if you don't invest now. Just like saving money in your piggy bank for your retirement, eating healthy raw fruits and vegetables is essential for your future health. The reward and investment returns are that you will have more energy, sleep better, be more focused, feel healthier, look younger, have beautiful skin, and you will not bankrupt your family with medical bills. In addition, you will be doing your part to keep the healthcare industry from bankrupting the government and our country.

Chapter 2

HOW THE BODY USES NUTRIENTS

Don't dig your grave with your knife and fork.
– English Proverb

Our body is an amazing machine that has the ability to create and heal us. In my profession, we say, "The power that makes the body, heals the body." This incredible machine has the ability to produce all the drugs in the drugstore plus more without any side effects, it regenerates new cells, and it gets rid of toxins without us realizing or noticing it. The body has such an efficient system that science cannot replicate it.

So how does this incredible machine use vitamins and minerals to build a healthy body? Our body uses different vitamins and minerals to produce different functions. Take for example how our body needs manganese and iron to produce healthy black hair. A diet low in manganese-rich raw vegetables will lead to a deficiency that not only contributes to gray hair but also inflammation, joint pain, arthritis, diabetes, and epilepsy.

The body is composed of 60-100 trillion cells, and according to scientist Stephen Cherniske, our body reproduces 300 billion cells daily. All the vital tissues in a healthy body are replaced every fourteen months and some tissues much more frequently while our bones are replaced every seven years. If our body produces 300 billion cells daily to replace older cells, but the replacement cells are weaker than the older ones due to poor nutrition, then optimal health diminishes and chronic disease begins. In other words, the health of new cells daily produced by our bodies is the direct result of what we put into our bodies on a daily basis.

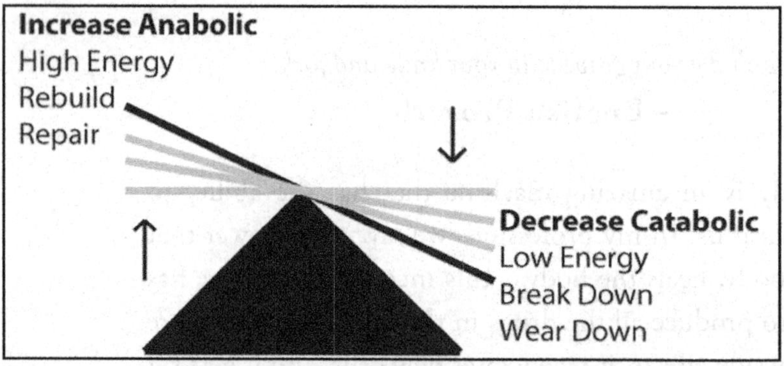

Courtesy of Stephen Cherniske, M.S.

The above diagram demonstrate that as we eat healthy foods rich in vitamins and minerals, our bodies use these materials to build newer and stronger cells like those in healthy children.

Think of a newborn baby. Consider the dramatic changes that babies go through in just a few days, weeks, and months. They grow and change most dramatically from birth to being one year old.

Here are some examples of my daughter, Faith:

These dramatic changes are the result of the nutritious foods babies are given which allow the body to regenerate 300 billion

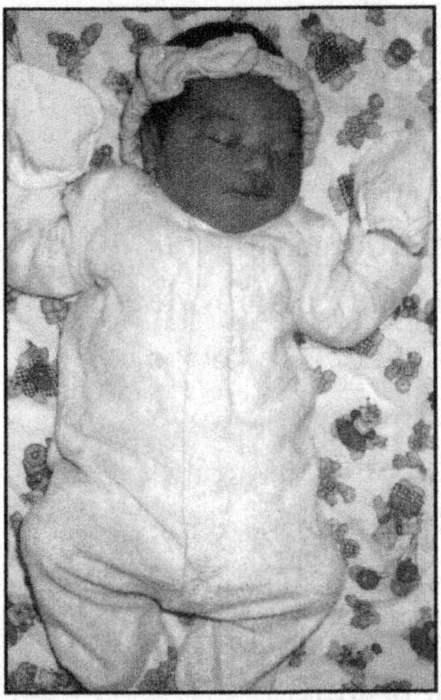

Two days old

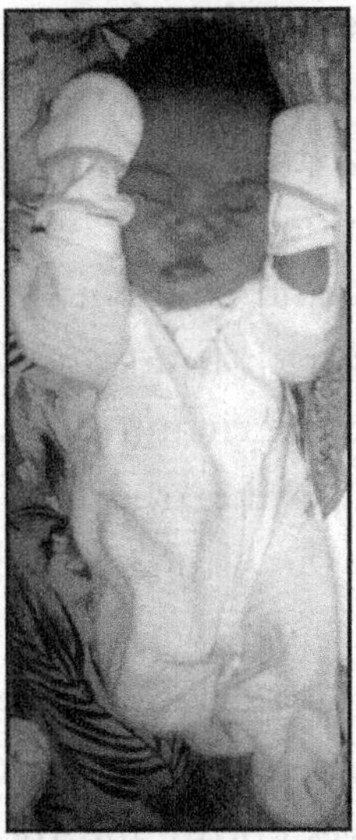

Two weeks old

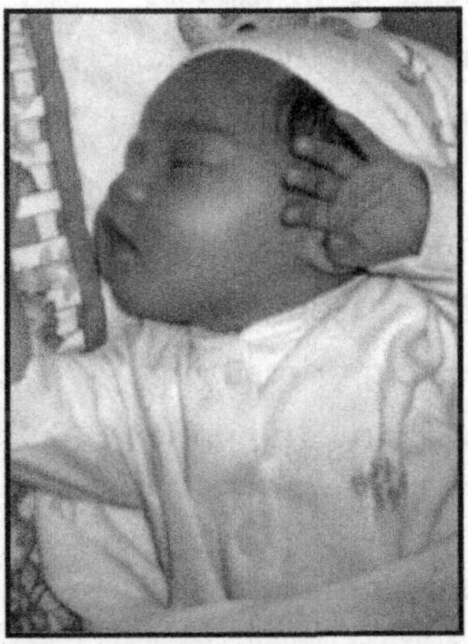

One month old

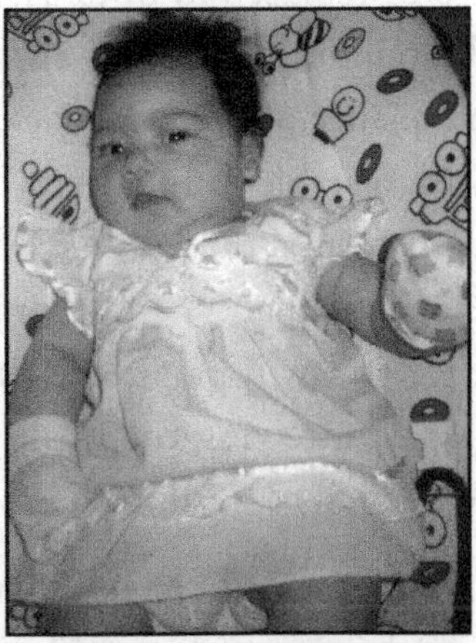

Two months old

new cells daily. And those cells are constantly replacing old cells with stronger, more vibrant ones.

Another great example of how good nutrition helps generate healthy new cells is Jack LaLanne, the "Father of Fitness." Jack is ninety-five at the time of this writing, but he's living life like he was in his twenties, and he looks like he's in his sixties. He has more stamina and endurance than most college students today. Jack juices fresh fruits and vegetables daily to provide his body with optimal vitamin and mineral intake. Jack knows that healthy food is the true foundation to a healthy body and that without this strong foundation, life and our health is simply filled with deficiency. And deficient nutrients are the cause of such chronic diseases as constipation, irritable bowel syndrome, obesity, hypertension, arthritis, and cancer. For that reason, Jack believes nutrition is the queen of health.

Our body uses vitamins, minerals, and essential oils to build strong new cells to replace old ones. As we learned in the last chapter, it's like building a home—the strength of the home depends on the quality of the materials we use to build it. We have to start with a stable foundation, or no matter the quality of the other materials, the house will be unstable. A master builder will recognize quality, but an unskilled person cannot tell the difference and will pay the asking price, not realizing that he may not be receiving the quality he wants. The same concept can be applied to our health.

For instance, when we eat green leafy vegetables that are rich in nutrients like calcium, our body uses them to our advantage. We all know calcium makes our teeth and bones strong, but it is also vital for a healthy thyroid to function. Calcium helps in making our blood clot, in metabolizing fat, regulating digestion, maintaining our phosphate balance, and it is vital in the production of numerous enzymes. Calcium is absorbed in our small intestine called the duodenum, and it requires vitamin D for it to be absorbed into the bloodstream, so it is critical that a sufficient amount of vitamin D is available if a sufficient amount of calcium is to be absorbed. Vitamin D is also needed to absorb phosphorus, to maintain healthy nerves and muscles, and to keep our bodies immune from disease. A vitamin D deficiency leads to osteoporosis and calcium deposits in soft tissues such as in the lungs, breasts, and kidneys (kidney stones). Calcium and vitamin D deficiencies also cause muscle cramps, high blood pressure, insomnia, arthritis, and tooth decay. Although our bodies may intake a large amount of calcium, without vitamin D, the body will not absorb it.

To get vitamin D, we need sufficient sunlight exposure, which depending on where you live can be easy or difficult. For example, in Seattle, our sunlight exposure is very limited.

We need to eat a balanced diet of fruits and vegetables rich in vitamins and minerals for our bodies to build stronger and newer cells. Our body functions like an amazing machine that works in ratio and systematic orders. According to scientist Paul Eck, the ratio of calcium (Ca+) to potassium (K+) should be 40/6 mg so the thyroid glands will function optimally. And a ratio of 25/10 mg of sodium (Na+) to magnesium (Mg+) is needed for optimal functioning of the adrenals glands. Lower ratio levels will affect the body's overall health, including its ability to produce energy and rebuild healthy cells.

What about potassium? We know potassium is needed for

muscle contraction, but it also plays many other vital roles in the body. A proper potassium and sodium ratio of 2:5 is essential to the body's balance of fluid for optimal health. Thus, a potassium deficiency can lead to many health risks such as stroke, hypertension, irritable bowel syndrome, and muscle cramps. Potassium is found in 1) green leafy vegetables like kale, cabbage, and broccoli, 2) fruits such as bananas, cantaloupes, and avocados, and 3) meat like salmon and cod.

Thus, if we eat unhealthy, non-nourishing foods, the body does not have the right raw materials to build the strong cells essential for a healthy foundation. For example, scurvy results from a vitamin C deficiency. Vitamin C, found in citrus fruits such as oranges and limes, is necessary to form collagens used by our bones, skin, organs, and tendons.

Recent research shows that a deficiency in essential vitamins, minerals, and essential oils causes immune weaknesses that result in such conditions as cancer, autism, diabetes, allergies, asthma, ADHD, MS, irritable bowl syndrome, stroke, obesity, eczema, hypertension, high cholesterol, depression, and many more. Our healthcare costs are so expensive now because of this fundamental nutrient deficiency in our bodies. If we make healthy choices about our daily food intake, we will see increased energy and the rebuilding and repairing of our cells. If we make unhealthy choices, we will see the opposite.

Failure to eat healthy foods so our bodies can have the proper nutrients makes us age more quickly, and for our children, it does not allow their bodies to develop properly. If we want to protect our children from suffering from obesity, diabetes, juvenile arthritis, and other diseases, we must provide them daily with the proper levels of nutrition especially in the form of raw vegetables and fruits to keep their cells strong and alive.

Decreased health is due to poor daily intake of nutrients combined with stress from lack of sleep, poor exercise, being overworked, financial hardships, etc. As indicated, when we are young a good source of nutrients is provided to us, but as we become adults, we tend to lose that source of nutrients due to poor eating choices. Today, we are beginning to see more rapid aging in younger children than we did thirty years ago precisely because their diets are so poor in nutrients that they are considered malnourished. Their bodies are breaking down faster than they can repair or rebuild themselves because a lack of nutrients leaves them nothing to build a foundation upon.

Another example of nutrients vital to the body is essential oils, often called fatty acids because they consist of long-chain polyunsaturated fatty acids derived from linoleic acids (omega-6), linolenic acids (omega-3), and oleic acids (omega-9), which the body needs and is unable to make. Essential fats are important for forming the structures of cell membranes and for producing hormones and steroids. Furthermore, both omega-6 and omega-3 play a major role in our overall health because they are involved in normal growth. Omega-6 is better at supporting skin integrity, renal function, and parturition, but it breaks down in the body faster than omega-3, so for omega-3 to compete with omega-6, our daily intake of omega-3 needs to be more than omega-6. Omega-6 needs to be balanced out with omega-3 because omega-6 also has negative effects such as increasing inflammations, blood clots, increased blood pressure, and oxidizing cholesterol, while omega-3 helps to suppress inflammations, lowers blood pressure, prevents blood clotting, prevents heart disease, forms soluble cell walls, benefits type-2 diabetes, decreases high blood pressure, prevents cancer and cardiovascular diseases, enhances immune functions, improves brain functions, and prevents arthritis. Thus, the recommended daily intake ratio of omega-6 to omega-3 should be between a 1:2 and 1:4 ratio. However, the Standard American Diet ratio is closer to between 10:1 and 30:1. Recent statistics show 97-99 percent of the U.S. population has a deficiency of omega-3, which is directly responsible for the increase in juvenile arthritis, diabetes, and hypertension. Omega-3 oils are known to help children with asthma, ADHD, autism, and psychiatric disorders.

Since both omega-3 and omega-6 can only be found in plant oils such as coconut, flaxseed, hempseed, walnut, pumpkin seed, avocado, dark green leafy vegetables, and in fish oils like salmon, tuna, mackerel, and sardines, eating the Standard American Diet provides the body with no nutritional value. A diet rich in omega-6 increases the chronic inflammation inside the body that leads to diseases like diabetes, arthritis, cancer, and asthma. Therefore, doctors and nutritionists recommend eating fish, nuts, fruits and vegetables to get the daily omega-3 essential oils necessary to counteract omega-6 and to build strong cells. Eating a balanced meal with everything in moderation is the key to creating a healthy life.

I recommend using coconut oils for all cooking and beauty applications on the skin. Coconut oils have antioxidant, antiviral, and anti-inflammatory components. Coconut oil contains medium-chain fatty acids that are easily absorbed into the body and help protect it against heart disease. Extensive research has also shown the health benefits of coconut oils for conditions like constipation, infection, stomach aches, the common cold, flu, seizures, liver disorders, and many more. Coconut oil is cheap, and it is healthy to stir fry with because high heat does not break its bonds as happens with canola, olive, and vegetable oils. For more details about the benefits of coconut oil, visit www.coconutresearchcenter.org.

No matter how much we try to focus on healthy eating, at times we all get off track, and due to the toxins in our environment, our body also needs added support. Two additional support supplements I highly recommend are enzymes and probiotics.

Enzymes are catalysts that help to break down food and make the body work faster. Enzymes are necessary for the day-to-day bodily functions of every organ system from digesting food to absorbing the nutrients we eat, eliminating toxins, and many more. Enzymes are usually produced within the body and include:

- **amylase** produced in the mouth to break down carbohydrates
- **pepsin and hydrochloric acid** produced in the stomach to break down proteins and aid in digestion
- **lactase** to break down milk sugar
- **DPP IV** to break down milk protein and other protein bonds
- **disaccharides** to break down starches and sugars in our small intestine

Although the body manufactures enzymes, their production may be limited or they may be lost due to leaky guts, inflammation, yeast, or other health issues that affect the small intestines.

Furthermore, if our diet is lacking in the fruits and vegetables that contain necessary enzymes, the body could become depleted from its natural production of enzymes. When our body is required to produce more enzymes to cope with the demand of the body's daily activity, the thyroid and digestive glands have to work extra hard to produce the necessary number of enzymes. When the body must overexert itself to produce enzymes so it can perform its daily functions, it causes enlarged and overworked organs and glands, which in turn lead to degenerative disorders like osteoporosis, gastrointestinal disorder, and Alzheimer's, and to auto-aggressive disorders such as lupus, rheumatoid arthritis, and cancer.

The role of enzymes is far more complex than what I have described here, but this brief introduction is sufficient to understand that a deficiency in enzymes can greatly compromise our health. According to scientists, alterations, defects, and an absence, insufficiency, or excess of enzymes can contribute to the creation of diseases. Therefore, to make sure you are getting a sufficient number of enzymes, eat fruits and vegetables at every meal. Organic produce especially rich in enzymes includes Brussels sprouts, pineapple (rich in the enzyme called bromelain), and papaya (rich in the enzyme called papain). You can also take a plant enzyme supplement with every meal if you are not eating enough fruits and vegetables.

Probiotics are the good bacteria in our guts. Since 80 percent of our immune system is in our gut, it is important to make sure we have a sufficient amount of good bacteria there to combat bad bacteria, yeast, and fungus. This good bacteria also helps to increase absorption of calcium in the bloodstream, to produce vitamin B, to support the liver's function, to support cholesterol management, and to balance our bowel movements. Overprescriptions of antibiotics can destroy good bacteria, making a probiotics supplement essential. Supplements such as Lactic Acid Yeast, Kombucha drinks, and Bragg Organic Raw Apple Cider Vinegar are all designed to help replenish the intestinal flora. In my years of practice, I found that patients with chronic inflammation and intestinal tract disorder greatly benefited from a combination of enzymes and probiotics when used on a daily basis.

Below, I have compiled a list of vitamins and minerals, their benefits to the body, the recommended daily allowance (RDA), bodily symptoms that result from their deficiency, and food sources for them. Remember that our body requires daily moderation and balance of different vitamins and minerals to build a healthy body that can function at its optimal level. Eating a variety of fruits, vegetables, nuts, and meat will provide the different nutrients your body needs. Also remember that no two human bodies are the same so by understanding the benefits derived from each vitamin or mineral, hopefully, you will be compelled to try different ones to determine how to meet your body's nutritional requirements.

VITAMINS:

- **Vitamin A:** Good for vision, immune function, cell reproduction, bone growth, skin health, red cell production, and cancer prevention

  RDA: 5000 IU (International Unit)

  Signs of Deficiency: Blindness, increased respiratory infection, and decreased immune functions

  Sources: Yellow, orange, and green leafy vegetables, sweet

potatoes, eggs, and cod liver oil

- **Vitamin B1 (Thiamin):** Helps to break down blood sugar into energy; protects against alcoholism; is vital to the nervous system; increases mental ability; aids cardiovascular and muscular function; helps digestion; and relieves depression, stress, and anxiety

  RDA: 1.2-1.5 mg

  Signs of Deficiency: Beriberi disease (a muscle-wasting condition), confusion, nerve problems, rapid heartbeat, muscle weakness, nausea, loss of appetite, constipation, irritability, and depression

  Sources: Brown rice, sunflower seeds, oatmeal, pork, and peas

- **Vitamin B2 (Riboflavin):** Manufactured in the body by good bacteria. Essential for metabolizing carbohydrates, fats, and proteins needed to activate vitamin B6; helps adrenal glands; helps formation of red blood cells; provides antibody production; helps cell respiration and cell growth; prevents and treats cataracts; protects against cancer; and helps to produce healthy nails, hair, and skin

  RDA: 1.7 mg

  Signs of Deficiency: Dizziness, insomnia, poor digestion, retarded growth, slow mental response, burning feet, hair loss, and chronic fatigue

  Sources: Leafy green vegetables, almonds, and free range eggs

- **Vitamin B3 (Niacin):** Helps to detoxify the body; metabolizes carbohydrates, proteins, and fats into energy; assists in GI functions; promotes normal appetite; and helps to produce healthy skin and nerves

RDA: 13-18 mg for adults, 9-13 mg for children

Signs of Deficiency: Weak muscles, indigestion, loss of appetite, memory problems, tiredness, and skin problems

Sources: Usually found in meat, eggs, and nuts

- **Vitamin B5 (Pantothenic acid):** Boosts energy production by metabolizing carbohydrates and fat; increases muscle metabolism; aids in hormone production; assists in healthy brain functions; boosts fat metabolism; maintains hair, skin, and nails; lowers cholesterol; and helps to relieve stress

  RDA: 10 mg

  Signs of Deficiency: Low energy, irritability, fatigue, paresthesia, and poor concentration

  Sources: Green leafy vegetables, oats, free range eggs, meats, and nuts

- **Vitamin B6 (Pyridoxine):** Boosts immune system; metabolizes fats, proteins, and carbohydrates into energy; serves as a coenzyme for many reactions in the body; helps with skin and nervous disorders; helps with morning sickness, anti-aging properties, anti-cancer properties, histamine synthesis, hemoglobin synthesis, and the function of gene expression; essential in detoxification

  RDA: 2 mg

  Signs of Deficiency: Skin disorder, conjunctivitis, depression, poor ability to detoxify chemicals, loss of appetite, irritability, and being more prone to infection

Sources: Free range eggs, oats, mackerel, meat, avocado, banana, brown rice, and cabbages

- **Vitamin B7 (Biotin):** Promotes cell growth and production of fatty acids; metabolizes fats, proteins, and carbohydrates; strengthens nails and hair

  RDA: 300 mcg (microgram)

  Signs of Deficiency: Conjunctivitis, alopecia, depression, anorexia, numbness and tingling, poor appetite, and fatigue

  Sources: Free range eggs, oatmeal, peas, mackerel, avocado, and brewer's yeast

- **Vitamin B9 (Folic Acid):** Essential for the synthesis of DNA and for the growth and maintenance of all cells; involved in production of neurotransmitters that regulate mood, sleep, and appetite; prevents heart disease; and reduces homocysteine levels in the blood

  RDA: 400 mcg

  Signs of Deficiency: Loss of appetite, weight loss, cracked lips, anemia, and depression

  Sources: Orange juice, spinach, lentils, asparagus, and rice

- **Vitamin B12 (Cyanocobalamin):** Plays key role in normal functioning of brain and nervous system; metabolizes proteins, fats, and carbohydrates into energy; used to regenerate folate in the body

  RDA: 6 mcg

Signs of Deficiency: Fatigue, depression, poor memory, anxiety, eczema, and pale complexion

Sources: Meat, free range eggs, and fish

- **Vitamin C (Ascorbid Acid):** Antioxidant; an enzyme cofactor for collagen formation; promotes healthy teeth, gums and bones; strengthens connective tissue healing; detoxifies chemicals

  RDA: 60 mg

  Signs of Deficiency: Poor immune function, bleeding gums, bruising easily, nose bleeds, slow wound healing, and scurvy if severe

  Sources: Rose hip, red pepper, broccoli, parsley, and guava

- **Vitamin D:** Regulates absorption of calcium and phosphorus; maintains healthy nerves and muscles

  RDA: 400 IU

  Signs of Deficiency: Muscle cramps, tooth decay, hair loss, joint pain, and decreased immune functions

  Sources: Salmon, tuna, free range eggs, cod liver oil, mackerel, and mushrooms

- **Vitamin E (Tocopherol):** Antioxidant; protects cell membranes from oxidation; prevents cancer and heart disease

  RDA: 30 IU

  Signs of Deficiency: Varicose veins, abnormal tiredness after exercise, slow healing of wounds, and reduced sex drive

  Sources: Olive oil, almonds, hazel nuts, avocados, and sunflower oil

- **Co-Enzyme Q10:** Antioxidant; improves heart functions; lowers blood pressure; improves immune functions

  RDA: Not established

  Signs of Deficiency: Heart disease and poor immune function

  Sources: Hazel and pistachio nuts, mackerel, cabbage, carrots, and spinach

Minerals:

- **Calcium:** Development and maintenance of healthy bones and teeth; aids in blood clotting; metabolizes fat; essential in production and activity of numerous enzymes and hormones that regulate digestion

  RDA: 1000 mg

  Signs of Deficiency: Muscle cramps, high blood pressure, arthritis, insomnia, and tooth decay

  Sources: Spinach, black eyed peas, yogurt, whole milk, cottage cheese, and almonds

- **Iron**: Transports oxygen in blood to all parts of the cells; improves immune functions; essential for energy production

  RDA: 18 mg

  Signs of Deficiency: Breathlessness, anemia, pale skin, sensitivity to cold, loss of appetite, nausea, low energy

  Sources: Lean red meat, seafood, beans, and green leafy vegetables like kale, broccoli, and asparagus

- **Magnesium:** Metabolizes fats, proteins, and carbohydrates for energy; vital in the production of ATP, DNA, and RNA; used as a laxative; improves nerve transmission; strengthens bones and teeth; promotes healthy heart and limbs

RDA: 400-420 mg for adults

Signs of Deficiency: Tremors, muscle spasms, insomnia, weak bones, headaches, depression, confusion, lack of appetite, irregular heartbeat, Crohn's disease, celiac disease, and diabetes mellitus

Sources: Spinach, pumpkin seeds, beans, artichoke, nuts, and buckwheat flour

- **Potassium:** Maintains normal balance of fluids throughout the body; maintains optimal blood pressure, calcium balance, and heartbeat; regulates nerve transmission and many cell membrane functions

  RDA: 4500 mg

  Signs of Deficiency: Irregular heartbeat, diarrhea, low blood pressure, confusion, pins and needles sensations

  Sources: Spinach, kale, mustard green, broccoli, cantaloupe, and turmeric

- **Selenium:** Antioxidant; reduces inflammation

  RDA: 70 mcg

  Signs of Deficiency: Premature aging, high blood pressure, cataracts, nerve degeneration, stroke, and anemia

  Sources: Halibut, salmon, eggs, sunflower seeds, and oats

- **Zinc:** Antioxidant; metabolizes fats, proteins, and carbohydrates into energy; speeds up the healing process; protects against sunburn; helps maintain healthy teeth, hair, and bones

RDA: 8-11 mg for adults

Signs of Deficiency: Growth retardation, diarrhea, infection susceptibility, poor immune function, frequent infections, acne, greasy skin, depression, loss of appetite

Sources: Spinach, sea vegetables, basil, thyme, pumpkin seeds, beef, and broccoli

In conclusion, it is obvious that nutrition plays a vital role in our body's health. Therefore, choosing to eat organic fruits, vegetables, and meats is the first small step to investing in your health. Choosing to create a healthy life for your family and yourself by investing a little bit more money into buying healthy foods compared to fast foods that are cheap and convenient will allow you to reap the investment payoffs of feeling healthier, stronger, thinner, more energetic, better rested, and looking younger. Conventional packaged foods and fast foods may appear cheaper, but they are deficient in the nutrients our bodies need. Plus, when you factor in the health risks they pose, you will be costing your body and your family more money in the long run than if you practiced healthy eating habits now. Furthermore, two homemade healthy meals for a family of four will only cost about $13.00 while two fast food meals for four people is easily $40.00 or more.

And don't forget, as discussed earlier, the health issue is what has caused the greatest number of bankruptcies among American families and the largest assault on our economy. If you invest in healthy food, you'll have more money later to enjoy when you retire, and you'll be alive and in good health to enjoy it. As I always tell my daughter, "Whatever choice you make today, you will have to accept the consequences of that choice tomorrow."

EXERCISE

What are five foods you love to eat on a regular basis that are not healthy for your body?

____

____

____

____

____

What are five fruits and vegetables you love to eat?

____

____

____

____

____

What are five fruits and vegetables you have not tried but would not mind eating?

____

____

____

____

____

Chapter 3

WHERE TO FIND NUTRITIOUS FOODS

I am thinking of the onion again.... Not self-righteous like the proletarian potato, nor a siren like the apple. No show-off like the banana. But a modest, self-effacing vegetable, questioning, introspective, peeling itself away, or merely radiating halos like ripples

– Erica Jong, Fruits and Vegetables (1971)

Now that we know why it is so important to eat a lot of fruits and vegetables, where can we get them for a good deal?

Mother Nature has given mankind all the abundant nutrients needed to supply each and everyone of us on earth. Look around and see the vast bountiful supplies available to us. Our body needs water, fruits, vegetables, and proteins, and the earth is filled with all of them. After all, the earth is two-thirds water. As for foods, just look at coconuts. They are all over tropical places such as Hawaii, the Philippines, and parts of Asia. The coconut is Mother Nature's hidden secret fruit. Coconut juice is not only the best natural flavored drink without added refined sugar and coloring, but it is nourishing as well. Coconut juice is like a natural Gatorade sports drink. Coconut meat is rich in omega-3 and fiber. An extensive amount of research has been done on the health benefits of coconut oil. It is known to help people lose weight, to aid in holding off Alzheimer's, and to lessen the likelihood or intensity of seizures. For more information about the benefits derived from coconuts, I recommend you read the book *Coconut Cures* by Bruce Fife, N.D.

Our civilization has advanced to make our lives more convenient, but our inventions that increase that ease—the electronic remote control, fast food restaurants, and computers we glue ourselves to daily—have also resulted in our health diminishing greatly. Thus, I recommend treating your family and yourself to food that will not only nourish your body but sustain it for many years to come.

Equipped with our knowledge of how the body uses the vitamins and minerals found in organic fruits, vegetables, and meats, we can go shopping with a grocery list of foods to nourish our bodies and strengthen our immune systems. These foods can be found in most grocery stores. For instance, where I shop, at Fred Meyer stores, there's a great organic section with reasonable prices. In the past, people who wanted good organic produce and meat had to travel to special grocery or co-op stores, but because of increased knowledge about the values of healthy eating, a high demand for organic fruits, vegetables, and meats has led to most grocery chains stocking these items.

Organic fruits and vegetables contain more nutrients than non-organic ones. Furthermore, food that is organic is not treated with toxic chemicals like pesticides to grow and process the produce. As for organic meat, it is raised on a farm where animals are treated humanely; they are allowed to run in the grass and eat the vegetation naturally designed for their bodies to digest. No growth hormones or antibiotics are given to the animals to make them grow faster so they can be slaughtered and sold more quickly. Organic products have green and white labels on them as illustrated below. The farmers who sell organic products must go through a process outlined by the U.S. Government in order to obtain these labels, which make the foods containing them very respectable and reliable.

USDA ORGANIC

Be selective. Foods are the first step in investing in your family's future health. If you don't want to pay out all of your life's savings to treat illnesses later, then start investing in healthy organic food now. It may be a little expensive to pay for organic fruits, vegetables, and meats, but it sure beats paying thousands of dollars in medical expenses later. Even if you spent your entire life's savings on medical treatments, it would not guarantee you would get back your health. The value of your health is priceless, so invest in it with all you can now to reap the fruits of your labor later in life.

Below, I have listed the top ten fruits and vegetables and top five herbs my children love to eat. They are all rich in nutrients and also phytonutrients which are anti-cancer and anti-inflammatory agents. For example, broccoli has phytonutrients called sulforaphanes that are known to decrease several types of cancer. You can get these fruits, vegetables, and herbs anywhere from your local farmer's market to a chain grocery store.

TOP TEN NUTRIENT-RICH FRUITS

1. **Avocado:** Rich in vitamins A, B, C, E, and K, folate, phosphorus, magnesium, fiber, and rich in essential fats.
2. **Berries (acai, blueberry, raspberry, blackberry):** Rich in antioxidants, calcium, magnesium, potassium, folate, fiber, and flavonoids.
3. **Coconut:** Rich in essential fats; an antioxidant, anti-fungal, and anti-viral; rich in vitamins, minerals, and fiber.
4. **Guava:** Rich in vitamins A, C, and K, folate, calcium, magnesium, potassium, phosphorus, essential fats, and fiber.
5. **Kumquat:** Rich in vitamin A, antioxidants, calcium, potassium, magnesium, phosphorus, essential fats, and fiber.
6. **Papaya:** Rich in vitamins A, C, E, and K, folate, potassium, fiber, carotenes, flavonoids, and enzyme papain.
7. **Passion Fruit:** Rich in vitamins A and C, phosphorus, potassium, magnesium, calcium, sodium, selenium, iron, folate, coline, fiber, and essential fats (high in omega-6 (968 mg) and a small trace of omega-3).
8. **Persimmon:** Rich in vitamin A, antioxidant carotenoid, potassium, calcium, fiber, and magnesium.
9. **Pineapple:** Rich in vitamins B and C, potassium, calcium,

essential fats, fiber, and enzyme bromelain.

10. **Pomegranate:** Rich in vitamins A, C, and K, antioxidants, fiber, potassium, phosphorus, folate, phytosterols, beta-carotene, magnesium, calcium, and protein.

TOP TEN NUTRIENT-RICH VEGETABLES

1. **Broccoli:** Rich in vitamins A, C, and K, folate, calcium, magnesium, potassium, phosphorus, essential fats (omega-3 and omega-6), protein, and fiber.
2. **Cabbage:** Rich in vitamins A and C, folate, calcium, magnesium, phosphorus, potassium, essential fats (omega-3 and omega-6), protein, and fiber.
3. **Carrots:** Rich in vitamins A, B, C, D, E, and K, biotin, calcium, potassium, magnesium, phosphorus, and antioxidants (alpha, beta, gamma carotenes, zeaxanthin, and xanthophyll).
4. **Cauliflower:** Rich in vitamins A, C, and K, choline, folate, potassium, sodium, phosphorus, calcium, magnesium, essential fats (omega-3 and omega-6), and fiber.
5. **Celery:** Rich in vitamins A, B1, B2, B6, and C, folate, tryptophan, manganese, phosphorus, magnesium, iron, calcium, and fiber.
6. **Green Mustard:** Rich in vitamins A, B6, C, E, and K, folate, manganese, calcium, potassium, and fiber.
7. **Kale:** Rich in vitamins A, C, and K, potassium, calcium, phosphorus, magnesium, sodium, folate, essential fats (omega-3 and omega-6), and fiber; contains phytonutrients called indoles which activate the liver enzymes to de-

toxify all toxins.

8. **Red Bell Pepper:** Rich in vitamins A, B, C, and K, folate, and fiber; rich in phytonutrients such as lycopene, lutein, and zeaxanthin.

9. **Snow Pea:** Rich in vitamins A, C, and K, potassium, phosphorus, folate, calcium, magnesium, sodium, and iron; rich in phytonutrients (beta carotene, lutein, and zeaxanthin).

10. **Spinach:** The vegetable that contains the most phytonutrients. Rich in vitamins A, B6, C, E, and K, calcium, iron, folate, and thiamin, riboflavin, magnesium, phosphorus, potassium, copper, manganese, protein, and fiber.

TOP FIVE HERBS & SPICES FOR COOKING

Tomatoes and oregano make it Italian;
wine and tarragon make it French.
Sour cream makes it Russian;
lemon and cinnamon make it Greek.
Soy sauce makes it Chinese; garlic makes it good.
— Alice May Brock

1. **Aniseed:** Rich in vitamins A, B, and C, calcium, potassium, phosphorus, magnesium, copper, zinc, essential fats (omega-6), protein, and antioxidants.

   Health Benefits: Anti-epileptic and anti-hysteric, anti-rheumatic, anti-septic, anti-spasmodic, aperient laxative, a carminative agent that reduces gas, decongestant, digestive, expectorant, insecticide, sedative, stimulant, and vermifuge.

*** Because anise oil has such a strong narcotic component, pregnant women should avoid using it. In cooking, use only a small amount to add aroma and derive health benefits.

2. **Garlic:** Rich in vitamins A and C, calcium, phosphorus, selenium, magnesium, protein, and essential fats.

   Health Benefits: Helps with common colds (increases immune fx), cancer (blocks cancer cell formation), heart disease (lowers cholesterol and reduces chance of plaque formation), hypertension, infection, and impotence.

3. **Ginger:** Rich in vitamins B, C, and E, calcium, magnesium, manganese, potassium, selenium, protein, and iron.

   Health Benefits: Helps to prevent ovarian cancer, colon cancer, morning sickness; reduces pain and inflammation, heartburn, common cold and flu, migraines, menstrual cramps; prevents diabetic nephropathy; helpful in blocking prostaglandin; anti-inflammatory properties; alleviates nausea.

4. **Lemon Grass:** Rich in vitamins A and C, calcium, folate, potassium, magnesium, phosphorus, manganese, essential fats, and iron.

   Health Benefits: Anti-fungal and anti-bacterial; a great cleanser (detoxifies the colons, kidney, and bladder); relieves spasms, muscle cramps, rheumatism, and headaches; contains anti-cancer properties.

5. **Turmeric:** Rich in calcium, magnesium, phosphorus, potassium, iron, antioxidant curcumin, and essential fats

(omega-3 and omega-6).

Health Benefits: Antiseptic, anti-inflammatory, anti-platelet activity, anti-bacteria, anti-cancer activity (especially when used with cauliflower has been shown to prevent and stop growth of prostate cancer); prevents breast cancer from spreading to lungs; prevents melanoma; reduces childhood leukemia; natural liver detoxifier; may prevent or slow Alzheimer's; natural pain killer and cox-2 inhibitor; aids in fat metabolism and weight management; reduces depression, boosts the effects of chemo drug paclitaxel and reduces its side effects; stops the growth of new blood vessels in tumors; speeds up wound healing.

*** Individuals with gallstones or bile obstruction should not use turmeric. And pregnant women should consult a family doctor before using it.

As you can see, these herbs have some of the most natural anti-bacterial and anti-inflammatory compounds in them. Because they are all natural, not only do they taste good in foods, but they nourish your body, prevent infections, and have no side effects. As an added bonus, these natural products cost far less than prescription medication or a visit to the ER. Using them provides another chance to make that little piggy bank investment I've been talking about. Each time you use one of these herbs, it's like dropping pennies into a piggy bank and then forgetting about them until the bank is full. When we eat these nourishing foods everyday, our body uses their nutrients to build stronger bones, cells, and increase our immune functions. The healthy properties of herbs do not get much publicity because they are natural and cannot be sold as drugs. We might call them Nature's best kept secret, but now that you are knowledgeable about them, use them to invest in your health.

As I said at the beginning of this chapter, Mother Nature knows best and for that reason has provided us with healthy organic fruits, vegetables, and herbs to make our bodies healthy and protect them from disease. Although chemicals and fast foods have replaced the old-fashioned homemade meal, with the knowledge you have gained, you can make better choices for your family and yourself.

Chapter 4

COOKING TIPS

I feel a recipe is only a theme,
which an intelligent cook can play each time with a variation.

– Madame Benoit

Cooking is actually very fun. I know a lot of my friends don't cook, and they are amazed by my cooking. Most of my friends were blessed with great moms to cook for them so all they had to do was study and get good grades. But my mom died during the Khmer Rouge regime, and in Asian culture, it is expected of young women to learn how to cook at an early age anyway. When I first started learning how to cook, I was a nervous wreck. I feared my dad would criticize me because as a traditional Chinese man, he was brought up with the expectation that all women should be great chefs, as well as loving wives who stayed home to take care of the family. How well a woman cooked reflected how much she loved her family.

My dad had me start cooking when I was still a sophomore in high school. I was very nervous when I first stepped into the kitchen. Trying to remember which ingredients go with which dish was intense. I remember asking my older sister to tell me all the ingredients for different kinds of stir fry and soup. I felt so overwhelmed, and it didn't help that my dad would joke about how he had to pay people to eat my cooking. But did you ever notice that when you face your fears head on, things just seem to fall in your favor? Well, that was what happened. Instead of memorizing every ingredient for every dish, I got down the basic ingredients and then I just added different vegetables to experiment with how I wanted each dish to taste. Gosh, that was a lot simpler than trying to remember different ingredients for each dish. I realized then that cooking is an art—you play around with different spices, pepper, salt, and various vegetables to create your own style. That's the difference between a chef and someone who just cooks. A chef creates his own recipe, while a cook just follows the recipe.

For those of you afraid of cooking, don't be. Trust me; if I can cook, anyone can cook! Cooking is easy. And you don't have my dad there watching your every move and criticizing you if it doesn't turn out right. So roll up your sleeves and enjoy cooking with me.

Every morning, I wake up an hour before my family so I can have a hot breakfast ready for everyone to eat before they go about their day. I believe anything in life, if we make an effort to do it, can and will be done. It is all a matter of priorities, and if you truly want to invest in your family's health, learning a few simple recipes will help you save money and also ensure you are eating healthy foods.

Here are recipes with variations for chicken broth and stir

fry that can feed a family of four each day of the week.

CHICKEN BROTH

There are two choices for making chicken broth:

1. Either boil the whole organic chicken in a large pot such as 16 quarts. Then cut off the amount needed and store the rest in the refrigerator.
2. Second, cut the organic chicken into four sections. Then cut each of the four sections into small portions and put them in Ziploc bags for future cooking.

Now use one of the sections and boil it with lemon grass in a 3.5 quarts pot.

- Fill the pot half full with water.
- Put the organic chicken into the water.
- Add one stalk of lemon grass with 2 tbsp. of sea salt (or more or less depending on your taste).
- Bring the water to a boil and then reduce the heat to medium for twenty minutes with covered lid. The broth should be very tasty once it is cooked.
- Now, you can add any kinds of vegetable you like. Add the vegetables while the cooked broth is still hot and then replace the cover so the vegetables will steam cook for a few minutes while you call your family to the table to eat.

STIR FRY

First, choose any kind of meat you want. I like to use organic ground beef.

- Turn on the heat to heat up the frying pan.
- Place 1 tbsp. of extra virgin coconut oil in the pan.
- Throw in a ½ lb. of ground beef and 1 tsp. of sea salt.
- Turn the heat down to medium and put a cover over the frying pan.
- Allow the meat to cook 5-10 minutes depending on how well done you want the meat.
- While the meat is cooking, peel ginger, and slice it thin to put into the stir fry.
- Also while the meat is cooking, wash up your vegetables for that day's menu.
- Once the meat is cooked, add your vegetables to the frying pan.
- Cover the lid and turn off the heat.
- The steam from the pan will cook the vegetables without destroying the nutrients.
- Wait a few minutes for the vegetables to steam and then serve.
- How about that? Seems pretty easy, huh? So let's start cooking! Here are my weekly menus:

MONDAY:

Chicken broth — Organic chicken, carrots, green mustard, ginger, and lemon grass.

Stir fry — Organic broccoli with ginger, ground beef, and sea salt.

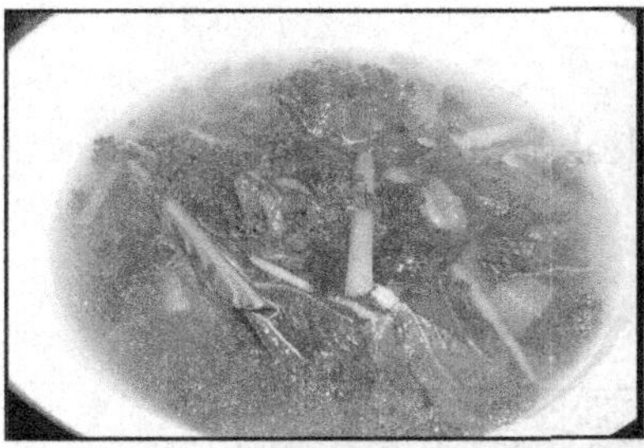
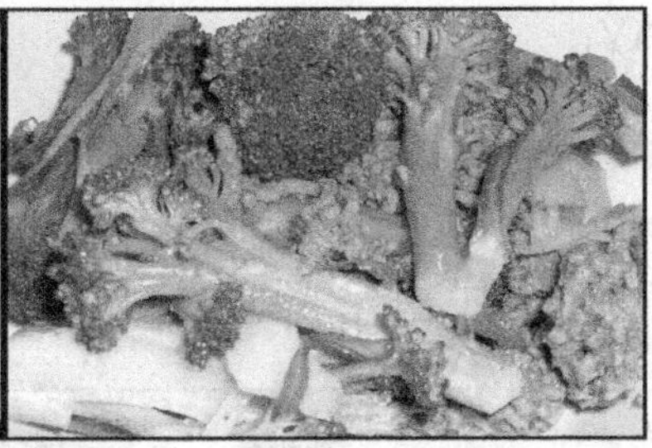

TUESDAY:

Chicken broth: Organic chicken, green collards, ginger, and lemon grass.

Stir fry: Organic ground beef, organic asparagus, parsley, ginger, and sea salt.

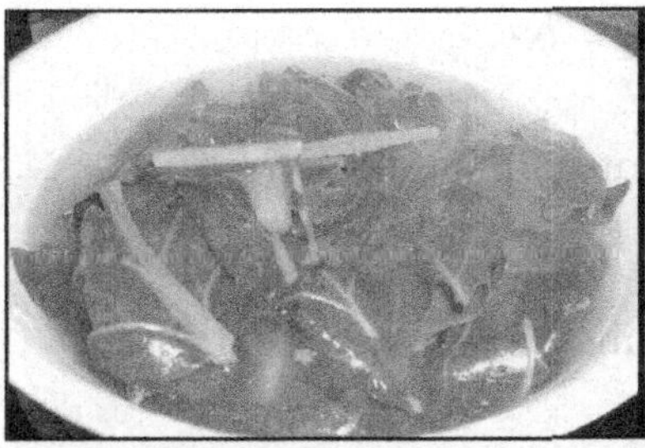
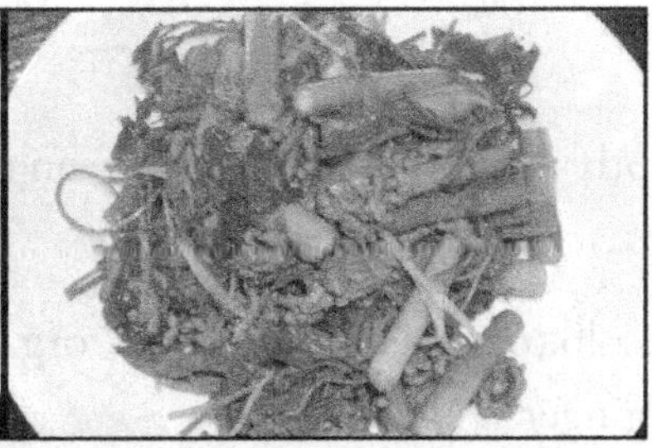

WEDNESDAY:

Chicken broth: Organic chicken, green mustards, ginger, and lemon grass.

Stir fry: Organic beef, organic celery, parsley, and ginger.

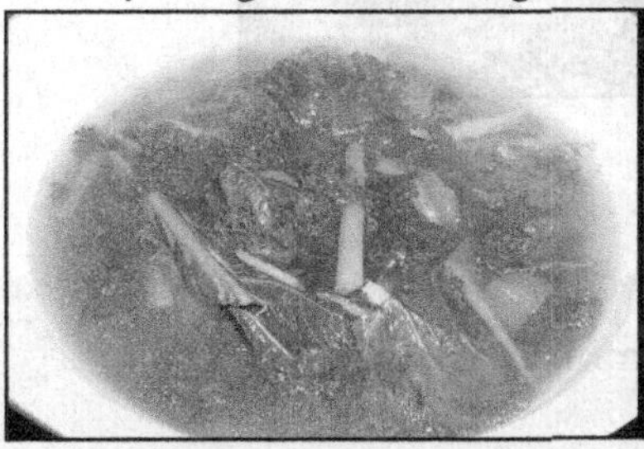
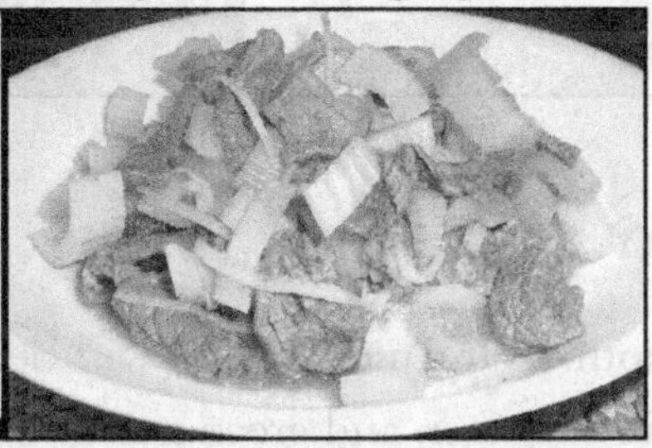

THURSDAY:

Chicken broth: Organic chicken, organic leaks, cabbage, ginger, and lemon grass.

Stir fry: Organic ground beef, chinese broccoli, and ginger

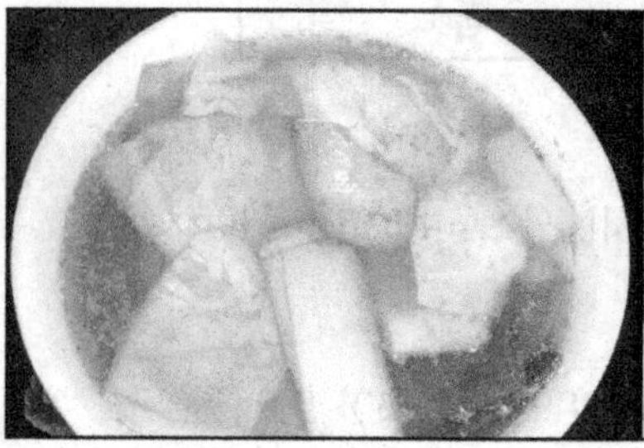
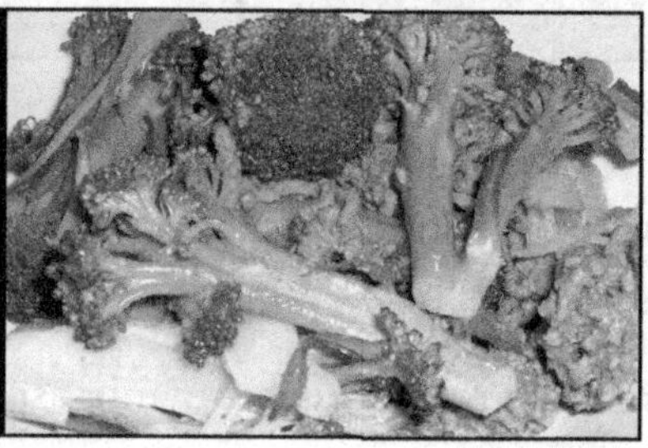

FRIDAY:

Chicken broth — Organic chicken, green mustard, ginger, and lemon grass.

Stir fry — ½ lb. organic ground beef, organic pineapples, turmeric, and ginger.

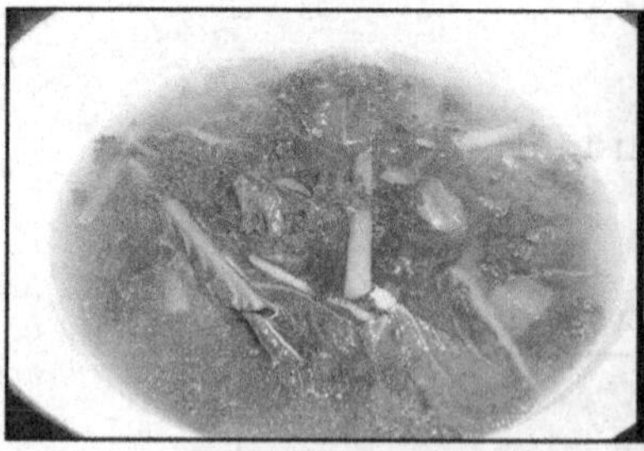
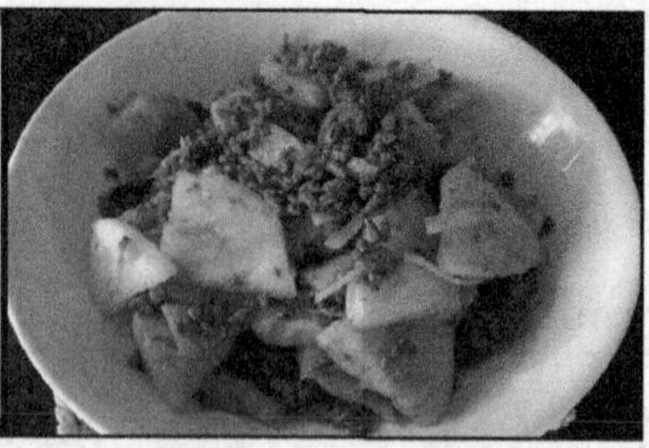

SATURDAY:

Chicken broth—Organic chicken with lemon grass, sea vegetables, carrots, ginger, and green mustard.

Stir fry—Grass fed beef and organic cauliflower with ginger.

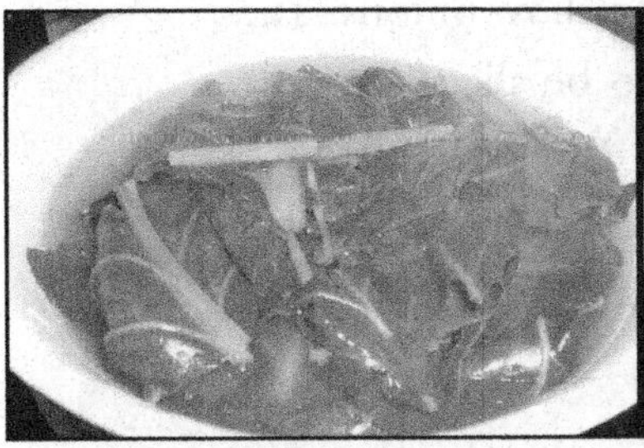

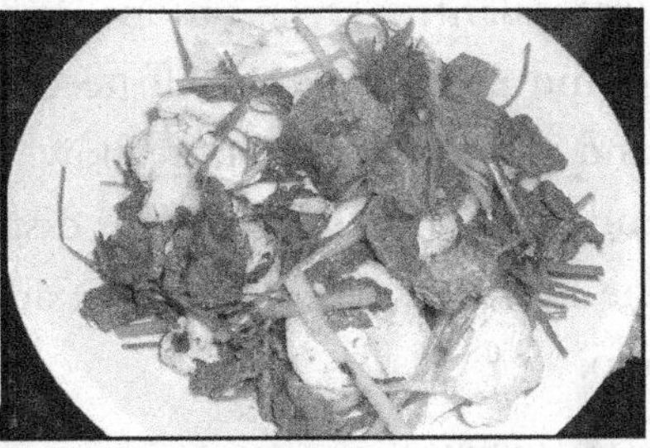

Step 1: Depending on the type of meat you like, you could use chicken, duck, or beef for the broth. The broth for the pho beef is simply cow bones, tendons, ginger, carrots, anise seeds (5 seeds), lime leaf (5 leafs), and 2-3 tbsp. of sea salt. Put all the ingredients into the 16 quarts pot and bring it to a boil. Once it boils, bring the heat down to medium and let it simmer for 3 hours. Allowing it to simmer is what makes a rich and delicious Pho broth.

As for using chicken or duck, put the whole chicken or duck into the 16 quarts pot and add slices of ginger, lemon grass, lime leafs (5 leafs), and 2-3 tbsp. of sea salt. Bring it to a boil and turn the heat down to medium.

Step 2: Soak the noodles for 5 minutes and rinse them into a strainer. Now, in a separate 3.5 quarts pot, fill the pot half full with water and then bring it to a boil. Just like when cooking spaghetti, once the water boils, put the desired amount of noodles into the boiling water and stir quickly until the noodles are cooked and soft. Then empty the pot into a strainer in the sink.

Step 3: Now that the noodles are ready and you have to wait for the broth to simmer, you can prepare the vegetables to add into the Pho. The vegetables are bean sprouts, basil, lime, cilantro, green onions, and yellow onions. The cilantro and green onions will need to be sliced up very small and put into a separate bowl. Add bean sprouts, lime, and basil to your taste. This dish is rich in nutrients from the fresh, raw vegetables you add on top of the hot Pho soup.

Bon Appetite!!!!!!!!

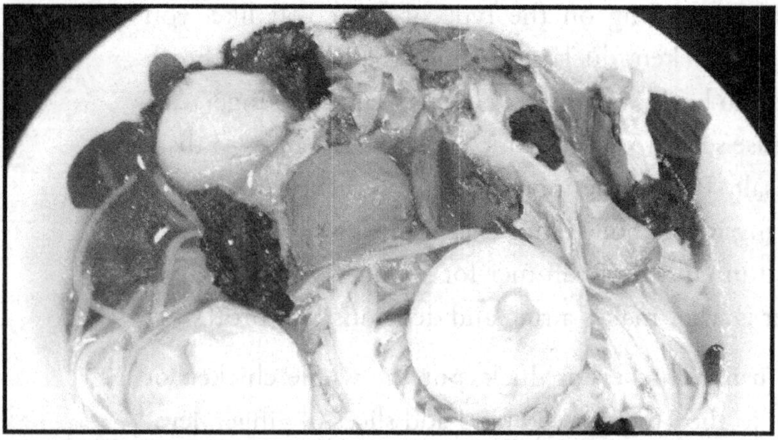

APPETIZER MENUS

Preparing appetizers is a great activity to do with your children. Here are two of my favorites: banana spring rolls and homemade fruit desserts.

Banana Spring Rolls:

Kids love to help make and to eat these. And they only take 10 minutes to prepare. You will need ½ pkg. spring roll wrappers, 5 ripe organic bananas, and extra virgin organic coconut oil.

First peel the bananas and cut them into 4 thin slices. Then peel the spring roll wrappers. Now put the sliced bananas into one corner of each spring roll and start to roll them. Seal them with egg yolks, or use corn starch glue if your child is allergic to eggs. While you are rolling the bananas, get a frying pan, add 1 cup of extra virgin coconut oil into the frying pan and turn on the heat to high. When the oil is hot, turn it down to medium and start to put the banana rolls into the frying pan. The banana rolls will cook very fast so turn them over when the bananas are golden brown to cook both sides. When the bananas are thoroughly golden brown, take the frying pan off the stove. Get a strainer and scoop the banana rolls out. Let them sit on a plate with paper towel underneath to soak up the oils. Serve them while they're still hot. They are great with ice cream!

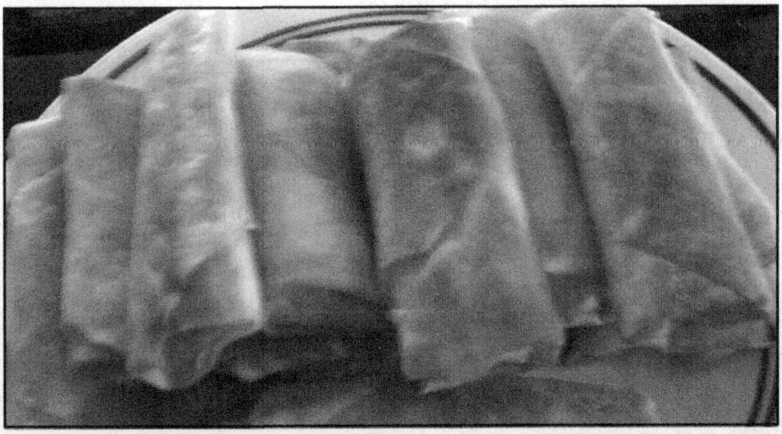

Homemade fruit dessert:

You can take the banana spring roll recipe above and modify it with different types of fruits. Once you have the basic steps to cooking down, cooking is fun and adventurous. It's actually an art. Be creative with the menus.

Cooking together and following these basic recipes is a great way for the whole family to enjoy a hot and nourishing, homemade meal. Now you will have nourished your whole family and may even have some leftovers to enjoy later. By eating homemade meals, you'll be able to spend quality time with your family. Recent studies show that if you spend family time together and eat together, your children are likely to do better in school and they will be better adjusted socially. And these homemade meals are easy to prepare. The average cooking time is simply 20 minutes. That's a small time investment when you consider the money saved, the benefits of eating nourishing and nutritious food, and the family time spent together.

Finally, here are two more of my top ten lists to help you know what to avoid and what to buy when you are in the grocery store looking for food to cook for your family.

TOP TEN HEALTH-LIMITING FOODS TO AVOID AND WHY

1. **Potato Chips:** Contain preservatives, MSG, high fats, high calories, high sodium.

   **** Fred Meyer's stores have a section of organic chips. If you must have chips, at least go for something healthier than the regular kind.

2. **Bacons:** Contain nitrite, nitrate, sodium, and MSG.
3. **Hot Dogs/Lunch Meats:** Contain nitrite, nitrate, high sodium, and MSG.
4. **French Fries:** Contain high sodium, high calories, and unhealthy oils.
5. **Donuts:** Contain a high number of calories, high fats,

and are loaded with refined sugars.

6 **Hamburgers:** Contain high fats, high calories, and MSG.

7. **Canned Soup:** Contain a high level of sodium and MSG.

8. **Fried Catfish:** Fried in trans fats.

9. **Soda:** High in sugar, caffeine, preservatives, and high in calories.

10. **Cold Stone Creamery Ice Cream:** Loaded with sugar and fat.

TOP TEN BEST FOODS FOR THE BUDGET CONSCIOUS

1. **Organic Eggs:** Rich in protein, essential fats, vitamins, and minerals.
2. **Organic Nuts:** Rich in proteins, essential fats, vitamins, and minerals.
3. **Fermented Beverages (Kombucha, Kefir):** Great for intestinal flora because they contain lactic acids and probiotics.
4. **Goat Products:** Easy to digest; rich in essential fats.
5. **Berries (all kinds):** Rich in anti-oxidants and are anti-inflammatory; rich in vitamins and minerals.
6. **Quinoa:** Rich in proteins, vitamins, minerals, and essential fats.
7. **Wheat Grass:** A good source of fiber and natural enzymes; loaded with vitamins and minerals.

8. **Seaweeds:** Rich in vitamins and minerals not found anywhere else; provide wonderful health benefits.
9. **Sweet Potatoes:** A great source of fiber, vitamins, minerals, proteins, and low in calories.
10. **Beans:** Rich in protein, vitamins B, and iron.

EXERCISE

What are five favorite dishes your family enjoys together?

What are five new dishes you think your family might enjoy?

Which of the five dishes above can result in the most family participation? (For example, my family enjoys spring rolls; everyone gets to make his or her own.)

Section 2

EXERCISE

Physical fitness is not only one of the most important keys to a healthy body; it is the basis of dynamic and creative intellectual activity.

–John F. Kennedy

Chapter 5

EXERCISE BENEFITS

A vigorous five-mile walk will do more good for an unhappy but otherwise healthy adult than all the medicine and psychology in the world.

– Paul Dudley White

As Americans become more and more obese, federal and state government officials are looking at ways to help solve this ongoing crisis affecting not only adults, but having a major impact on our children's lives. Obesity has affected over 72 million Americans and 16 percent of them are children. Obesity affects not just the physical aspect of life but also the psychological and social behavior of both children and adults. Children who are obese are more prone to hypertension, diabetes, heart problems, high cholesterol, cancer, liver and gallbladder disorder, and sleep apnea. Also, obese children have a shorter lifespan than adults as a result of these chronic diseases. Furthermore, 91 percent of obese children have type-2 diabetes, a direct result of lifestyle.

According to a study released by the World Health Organization (WHO), "physical inactivity is estimated to cause 2 million deaths worldwide annually. And 60% of the global population fails to achieve its minimum recommendation of 30 minutes a day exercise." Child obesity in America is on the rise as a direct result of a sedentary lifestyle, fast food, and refined carbohydrates.

The Centers for Disease Control are now looking at ways to address this epidemic by partnering up with state and local governments to implement a health plan to educate children about their health and to prevent childhood obesity.

First Lady Michelle Obama has decided to be the role model for millions of Americans and to tackle the deadly disease of obesity affecting millions of children by starting the "Let's Move" campaign. Mrs. Obama understands that we as parents and as a society have a responsibility for the future health of our children and their wellbeing. The first lady's campaign is named "Let's Move" because she understands how important it is to have children be more active and less sedentary. Mobilization and healthy eating are the key solutions to addressing the health issues resulting from obesity, and the first lady wants to educate parents and children both about the risks involved with obesity and how to prevent this deadly disease.

Recently, former President Bill Clinton, who had quadruple heart bypass surgery in 2004, was rushed to the emergency room in New York City's Presbyterian Hospital for chest pain. He has now joined California Governor Arnold Schwarzenegger for a health and nutrition summit to promote more exercise and a healthy lifestyle. Former President Clinton got a firsthand experience of how vital it is to invest in our health. He recognized the importance of proper sleep, exercise, and healthy eating. He is now committed to getting better sleep, exercising more, and eating more fruits and vegetables as a means to maintain his heart and overall health.

The benefits of exercise are becoming more popular and are more essential than ever before to our everyday stressful lives. More and more people are beginning to understand how exercise can greatly impact their health by providing them with pain relief and helping them to lose those extra pounds.

Do you know what the contestants on the reality TV show "The Biggest Loser" all have in common, besides being overweight? They have all tried to lose weight on their own, only to be unsuccessful. On the show, they succeed by having a personal trainer strip them of their regular Standard American Diet (SAD) and lazy couch potato lifestyle. The contestants then begin to lose weight for three reasons: 1) they no longer feed their bodies the junk food that causes them more harm, but replace that food with more nutritious fruits and vegetables to provide their bodies with the right material to build strong muscles and to adapt to new stress like exercise; 2) they exercise daily, which causes the body to stimulate the fat burning hormones to burn up more stored fats as energy; and 3) they give their bodies a break from all the toxins they consume on a daily basis and allow their bodies to remove the toxins they have had stored in them for years.

Toxins play a major role in our overall health, and exercise is king to removing toxins. I will elaborate more on toxins in Section Three, but I will mention toxins here where it relates to exercise.

Exercise has many benefits to our overall wellbeing beyond just losing weight. Losing weight is just one benefit from putting our body into motion again. Exercise brings motion to our body, which in turns gives us life. Our body is designed to be in motion, and without motion, we will die.

Look around. What do you see that is not moving and has life? Nothing!!! Look at the river that continues to flow to a never-ending site. Look at the birds that fly in the sky. Look at the waterfall with its magnificent power. Look at the flowers that bloom in the spring. Look at the clouds that change ever so constantly. Have you ever sat and listened to the flow of the water? There are immense life forces in the flow of water.

How about Mother Earth, which continuously spins around the sun without us even noticing its movement? All things in life have motion, and motion is life. Life without motion is death.

For that reason, our body was designed to be in motion, to move toxins out of our body, and to produce new cells so we can adapt to the constant change in our lives.

Our bodies are filled with moving life forces going on inside of us daily without us realizing it. Every part of our vital organs is playing its role in the motion of life. For example, the lungs are moving by squeezing our lung tissues in and out to get oxygen to supply the body. The heart is pumping blood in and out from our veins to our lungs to get fresh blood with oxygen and nutrients to all parts of our body. The GI tract is churning and grinding to get nutrients absorbed into the body and to eliminate waste. These life force movements are occurring every day. Our body works 24/7.

So if we decide to eat a lot of unhealthy foods, and then we come home and just sit around, watch television, play video games, or surf the Internet, eventually our body becomes sluggish and we gain weight. And the extra weight on our body stresses every part of our organs, especially the thyroid and adrenal glands. Worse, it makes us even lazier so when we do move around, we become easily tired. Laziness and obesity quickly become a vicious cycle.

Being lazy → sitting and watching television → gaining weight → decrease in energy → depression as a result of gaining weight → eating more to deal with depression → gaining more weight → joint pain caused from being overweight → more depression → eating → gaining more weight → being depressed → eating more → gaining more weight

Get the picture yet?

If this cycle goes on day after day, month after month, and year after year, it puts our health at risk for chronic diseases. Research has actually shown that office workers who make little effort to exercise are as at risk for health problems as people who smoke.

Most Americans don't exercise enough. They assume that work is exercise and that having a joint problem is a good excuse not to exercise. I believe the reason for most Americans' lack of exercise is a failure to understand the real need for exercise. Once more people understand why exercise is so vital, we will see more and more people out and about.

Thus, physical activity plays a major role in our overall health. Without it, we eventually die. Motion increases our metabolism by stimulating the fat burning hormones to burn fat, increase our mental clarity and focus, increase bone density, remove toxins, tone our muscles, strengthen our heart, improve circulation, grow new nerve cells, lengthen the life of cancer patients, and improve our vitality and youthfulness. Recent research has shown that exercise greatly benefits people with such chronic conditions as arthritis, asthma, diabetes, depression, obesity, stroke, osteoporosis, hypertension, fibromyalgia, chronic fatigue, and cancer.

Furthermore, exercise builds new muscle fibers by breaking down the old ones and making new ones, which is why we feel sore after a good workout. Also, exercise increases focus and improves overall body functions. Exercise also improves our brain functions because the brain is able to receive fresh blood that contains nutrients, and it is able to remove toxins through the blood-brain barrier. Also, if we don't exercise, the muscle fiber will waste away and cause degeneration of bones and nerve tissues as well; bones will become more fragile due to a decrease in calcium absorption. Studies show that by exercising, we increase our mental clarity, which in turn prevents us from getting Alzheimer's.

Exercise also helps our bodies to eliminate toxins. When we just sit around the house most of the time, then the body has limited motion which causes toxins simply to accumulate in our bodies. For millions of Americans who live with impaired digestion, lack of exercise increases their chances for bowel toxicity and toxicity overall in the body. Patients with Irritable Bowel Syndrome (IBS), Crohn's disease, or any other

GI conditions have a malfunction of their GI tract muscle and elimination mechanism. The constipation that results leads to a weak liver, weak kidneys, and weak intestinal linings with a decreased ability to absorb nutrients.

Accumulation of toxins → more disturbances to the elimination system → more accumulation of toxins → disease

Thus, conditions like depression, hypertension, arthritis, asthma, cancer, and diabetes can all greatly benefit from exercise. Exercise is effective because it works at our body's molecular level. Physical activity activates the body on a cellular level to release toxins and move nutrients into the cells.

Our bodies work 24/7 to remove toxins from our systems through five major organs: the lungs, liver, kidneys, large intestine, and the skin. Let's look at how each of these organs helps to remove toxins from our bodies and how that removal is heightened when we exercise.

THE LUNGS AND THEIR FUNCTIONS

Our lungs are designed to bring oxygen into the body and to remove toxins out through the mechanism of breathing. That is why breathing is so vital. Without air for even a few minutes, we would all die. The world record for holding one's breath is only seventeen minutes. The reason breathing is so integral to our lives is because when we take in a deep breath (inhale), we fill our lungs with fresh air rich in oxygen. When we breathe out (exhale), we release the toxins from our body. Our body uses the oxygen we inhale to turn it into the energy known as ATP so we can go about our daily activities. A lower degree of oxygen limits our ATP production, which puts our body in trouble because it will no longer have the power to remove toxins, keep us alive through the breathing mechanism, produce hormones, and perform all the other daily activities we ask of our bodies.

According to Dr. Fulford, "70% of our toxins such as carbon dioxides are eliminated through breathing." Breathing also helps to increase the body's overall energy level because it activates the cerebral spinal fluids produced in the brain which flow through the rest of the body. This fluid is the life force of our being.

Our body does not ask us to do much except to breathe, and it will do the rest. However, most of us are walking around taking very shallow breaths or practically holding our breath. Take a moment and observe your breathing right now. How are you breathing? Are you taking deep breaths in and out through your nose, or are you breathing rather slowly and with shallow breaths?

I catch myself holding my breath all the time. This is so bad! Why? Because every time you do not breathe fully, you are limiting the maximum amount of oxygen your body can intake, which retards your body's ability to be healthy. Since our body needs oxygen to produce energy, limited oxygen limits the body's ability to function. It's like shutting down the power, which is why without air, we would die.

THE SKIN'S FUNCTION

Another benefit of exercise is sweat which is the skin's way of releasing toxins from the body. The skin is a major organ system of our body that actually has many roles. It protects our body from harmful pathogens, it monitors and regulates our body temperature, it stores water and fat, and it can absorb, evaporate, and resist chemicals or water. But most importantly, it releases 20 percent of the toxins in the body through sweat. Therefore, exercise releases toxins. That's why you're told that when you exercise you should "work up a sweat."

THE KIDNEYS' FUNCTION

Our kidneys are amazing bean-shaped organs that are responsible for filtering waste and extra water. Each day the kidneys have to filter approximately 200 quarts of blood. The kidneys not only filter waste and extra water, but they are responsible for the regulation of blood pressure and maintaining the proper balance of electrolytes in our body.

THE LIVER AND LARGE INTESTINE'S FUNCTIONS

Other organs that play a role in removing toxins out of the body are the liver and the large intestine. The liver helps to filter most of the toxins in the body and then the large intestine carries out the elimination through bowel movements. Exercising helps keep the body in motion so we have regular bowel movements, which remove 7 percent of the toxins in our bodies. Failure to exercise leads to constipation and our body becoming one giant garbage landfill.

Imagine a landfill? Everything is dumped in the landfill until eventually it gets so full that another landfill is needed for dumping more waste, and on and on. You get the picture. In our body, when we continue day after day, month after month, and year after year to dump in tons and tons of toxins by eating unhealthy foods, drinking unhealthy beverages like sodas, breathing in unhealthy air from smoking and our toxic environment, and then not exercising, we are turning ourselves into landfills. The toxins find their way throughout all areas of our body, while our body is crying for help by giving us signs and clues it is in trouble in the form of pain like headaches, coughing, and constipation. If we ignore the warning signs and mask the problems by taking medication to hide the pain, soon the body can no longer eliminate the toxins and they spread to integral areas like the heart, liver, brain, and kidneys, causing those parts of the body to shut down. Patients diagnosed with such conditions as diabetes, arthritis, and cancer all had earlier signs and symptoms, but they chose to ignore them or did not know how to make changes to prevent diseases from forming.

Remember my earlier car analogy about how we know when to get more gas? Another car analogy is how we spend time taking care of our cars with regular oil changes, routine tune ups, and washing and cleaning them so they will last a long time. We want a reliable car because we paid an expensive price for it and we expect to get our money's worth. We all know that if we maintain our car, it will last us a long time and we won't have to fear it breaking down on us. Americans are masters at taking care of their cars; we need to give the same attention to taking care of our health.

Our body requires the same care as a car if not more. It requires regular tune ups, oil changes, and washes so it will last us for the many years to come. But for some reason, the concept that we need to take care of our bodies was not taught to us in school or anywhere. Instead we give it the wrong kind of fuel, fail to maintain it, and as a result, it eventually quits running.

When I was in college, I had no knowledge whatsoever about cars. All I knew was to put the key in to turn on the engine. One day, I had a final exam in inorganic chemistry very early in the morning. When I turned on my car, I noticed a red light come on. I had previously asked my brother to look at the car when the same thing had happened, but he had told me, "It's fine. It's an old car and the wire switch to the light is messed up." So I believed him and drove with the red light on. But that morning, as I was about to turn up the hill to the school entrance, my car's engine stopped. Frantically, I managed to get a passerby to help me push the car to the side of the hill so it was out of the way of oncoming traffic. Then I ran up the hill to ask my chemistry instructor to give me a chance to take the final exam, even though I was late. After I finished my exam, I asked my brother to look at my car. When he couldn't figure out what was wrong with it, I asked my dad to come take a look at it. It turned out that one of the wires was severed.

The moral of the story is that our body communicates with us all the time. It gives us a signal every time something is not right, but because we are trained not to listen to our bodies, we tend to ignore the signs and symptoms until it is too late. For example, I have patients who tell me their pain is just the normal result of old age, but it is not aging that causes you to feel pain—it's something else like a deficiency of nutrients, and the pain is the body's warning that it needs help. With my car, I ignored the sign, only to pay the price when the car broke down. When our body gives us signs, such as pain, being tired, or being constipated, we need to pay attention and correct the problem before our body breaks down. For instance, a migraine headache might be due to birth trauma, dehydration, or low blood sugar because you skipped a meal. Low energy can be the result of our body's thyroid and adrenal glands being overstressed or deficiency in minerals. By understanding how to listen to our body, we can address the problem early on before we have to pay the expensive price of neglect.

Exercise also requires us to drink more water. Our body is composed of 70-80 percent water, and that water needs to be replenished, yet many of us go all day drinking little to no water. If I were to poll Americans on how much water they drink, the average would probably be three or four glasses of water per day. Most believe that amount is a lot of water. Whenever I ask my patients if they drink water, I hear, "Oh yeah! I drink a lot!" But when I ask how many glasses they drink per day, the response is almost always three or four glasses. Some will even say, "I don't like water." We are so addicted to flavored drinks that water has become bland to our taste buds.

What most of us fail to realize is that water plays a vital role in our health. Water not only suppresses the appetite and helps our bodies to metabolize fat, but it regulates our body temperatures, transports nutrients and oxygen throughout the body, carries waste products away from the cells, cushions our joints, and protects our vital organs and tissues. Because our body is composed of 70-80 percent water, all of our vital organs, even the brain, is mostly water. According to Dr. F. Batmanghelidj, "many chronic degenerative illnesses can be prevented and treated with water." In his book *Water Cures*, Dr. Batmanghelidj talks about how water can help to cure diabetes, hypertension, lower back pain, acne, angina, migraine, colitis, high cholesterol, chronic inflammation, and many more ailments.

Remember how I mentioned during my senior year in high school I had severe acne? I tried everything from doctor prescriptions to washing my face three to four times a day with Clinique products. But what no one told me was that acne was a result of not drinking enough water. My body was crying for water! I had no idea I needed to drink more water and that my body was crying out for it. That summer when I decided to exercise more, I also drank more water, only to be pleasantly surprised when my acne started to disappear.

The majority of Americans are dehydrated, yet they continue to choose soda, coffee, juice or energy drinks over water as their daily intake of fluids. These beverages have little to no nutritious value and actually do harm to our bodies. For example, the caffeine in coffee and soda causes our kidneys to work harder to filter out the chemicals, thus increasing the need to urinate, which only causes the body to lose water faster. The body knows caffeine is a drug. In his book *Caffeine Blues*, Dr. Stephen Cherniske talks about how caffeine is the silent killer. He also says that caffeine speeds up our aging process. So for those of us who want to look young, coffee and soda are a "No, no." Furthermore, caffeine depletes our body of its energy, especially in the brain.

Therefore, water is the best choice. Not only is it cheap, but it provides healing effects for our bodies. When we exercise, we not only replenish our body with adequate amounts of water, but we also release toxins from the body, leaving us feeling happy, healthy, and energetic. Everyone should drink half of his or her body weight of water in ounces. So for example, if you weight 180 lbs, you should drink 90 oz. of water per day. Drinking that amount of water will allow the body to maintain its hydration level and will help all the vital organs to maintain their optimal functions.

Sleep is another great benefit of exercise. Sleep deprivation affects our overall health because it weakens the immune system, leaving us more susceptible to diseases and disorders like diabetes, cancer and even the common cold. Children who don't get enough sleep tend to be moody and cranky. They also have a poor time concentrating at school. Sleep also affects our body's ability to burn fat. Thus, if you want to lose weight, getting eight hours of beauty sleep will do you good. Plus, having a good night's sleep can save lives—every year over 100,000 car accidents and 1,500 deaths occur as result of fatigued drivers.

What causes us to lose sleep? Some of the key reasons are:

- Work: Working the swing or graveyard shift.
- Sickness: Inability to sleep due to the common cold, flu, fever, or cough.
- Environment: Living in noisy places, such as near highways, or near construction sites.
- Medication: Some medicines, especially for seizures and ADD, cause insomnia.
- Newborn children: Having a new baby in the house is exciting but also exhausting; when it doesn't sleep, neither do you.
- Choice: Choosing to stay up late surfing the Internet, or just hanging out or partying with friends.
- Stimulants: Drinking coffee, soda, or other caffeinated beverages in the evening.

To treat insomnia, exercise in the late afternoon or at least three or four hours before bedtime. When we exercise, our body temperature goes up and then gradually cools down. The cooling down of our internal temperature helps us to fall asleep more quickly. A research study by the Stanford University School of Medicine showed that when insomnia patients were asked to exercise twenty to thirty minutes a day in the afternoon, either by walking or by low-impact aerobic exercise, the time it took for patients to fall asleep was reduced by half.

What is the proper amount of sleep necessary for the body to maintain optimal health? On average, for children ages five to twelve, it should be ten or eleven hours, and for adults, it should be a good eight hours. The "Rule of Eight" is a good way to maintain health—eight hours of sleep and eight glasses of water. Going to bed early is also recommended. In our home, everyone is in bed by 8 p.m. When the children sleep, the adults also sleep. This allows me to get up early to make a hot breakfast for everyone. More importantly, going to bed early helps the body rejuvenate itself because the peak of Melatonin production is between 10 p.m. and 2 a.m. Melatonin is a hormone responsible for many functions in the body. One function is it helps our moods. That is why when children and adults get enough sleep, yawning, and the cranky, grouchy emotions are gone, and everyone is better able to focus at work and school.

Better muscle tone is the last benefit of exercise. Toning our muscles increase our body's metabolic rate for burning fat to use as fuels.

Research has proven that exercising just thirty minutes every day will improve a person's overall health, prolong lifespan, and sometimes cure illness and health conditions. All in all, exercise energizes every living cell in our bodies through the process of metabolism. Exercise increases metabolism, which converts glucose and oxygen into energy so our body can move and can build new cells.

So the second investment you need to make into your health is to exercise. Just as we invest money into maintaining our cars, we should invest thirty minutes everyday into exercise so we can achieve optimal health.

Exercise should be a joyful activity now that you understand all of its benefits. There should be no more excuses like:

- I am tired.
- I don't have the time.
- I am exercising when I am at work.
- My condition is too painful that I can't workout.

I challenge you the next time you exercise to do it with the intention not only to lose weight but to help your body clean out the toxins from every single cell. When our body is free from toxins, we feel good from the inside and we look good on the outside. Look at Jack LaLanne, the Father of Fitness. He is still going strong at ninety-five years of age. Young and old alike have wanted to know Jack's secret. The true secret to longevity, youthfulness, and good health is exercise and healthy eating. Get started doing both today!

EXERCISE

What is your favorite morning workout routine?

What are three things that keep you energized?

What family activities tend to get all of your family involved?

Chapter 6

TYPES OF EXERCISE

There are many different ways to exercise. The key to exercising is simply to keep your body moving. You can be gardening, swimming, jogging, walking, hiking, etc. As long as you are moving and doing something, then you are exercising.

Three of the most popular forms of exercise today which I will discuss in detail are: stretching exercises, aerobic exercise, and anaerobic exercise. All these exercises have their benefits.

STRETCHING EXERCISES

Stretching exercises include Yoga, Pilates, and Tai Chi. They are usually slow, and tolerable for the majority of people in all age groups. Stretching is the best type of exercise for senior citizens and patients with chronic pain because it does not require vigorous movement.

Stretching helps your muscles to become more lean and flexible. Flexibility and agility are a sign of youthfulness. Stretching also helps to break down adhesions and remove toxins like lactic acids out of the spastic muscles.

Stretching is an innate natural response seen in all animals. Look at dogs and cats in your home. When they get up in the morning, they stretch first before they go do their routine outside. I actually feel much better throughout the day when I get a good stretch in the morning. On days when I forget to stretch, I feel achy and stiff like a brick. Below are some of my favorite stretches I practice daily and recommend to my patients.

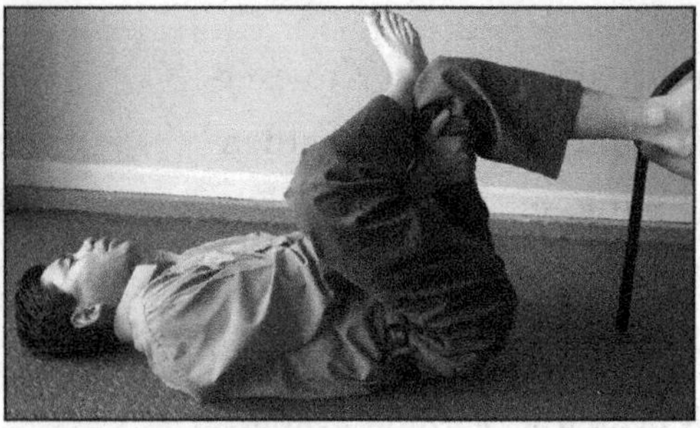

Piriformis Stretches: Great for patients with low back pain and low extremity conditions.

Lie on the floor next to a sofa and cross one leg over the opposite knee.

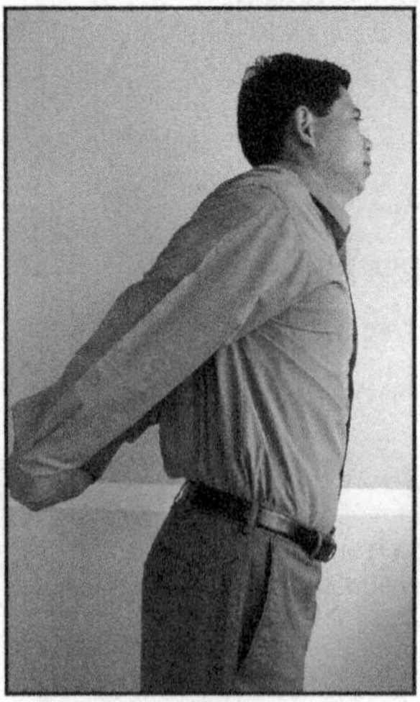

Bring the knee up and place the foot on the sofa. The closer you are to the sofa, the more stretch you will get. Hold a good thirty to forty seconds, let go, and repeat for ten sets.

Pectoral Muscle Stretches: Great for head forward posture, or for patients who sit in front of the computer a lot.

Stand straight up and interlock your hands behind your back and then raise them up as high as you can. A good stretch for your pectoral muscles is when you can bring your arms up to be level with your chest area.

Another option is to stand before an open doorway and place both hands on each side of the door frame. Push your chest forward and hold for forty seconds. Then move your hands up the door frame in four-inch increments to give a stretch to different areas of your pectoral muscles.

Hamstring Stretches: Great stretches for patients who sit a lot or patients with low back or knee problems.

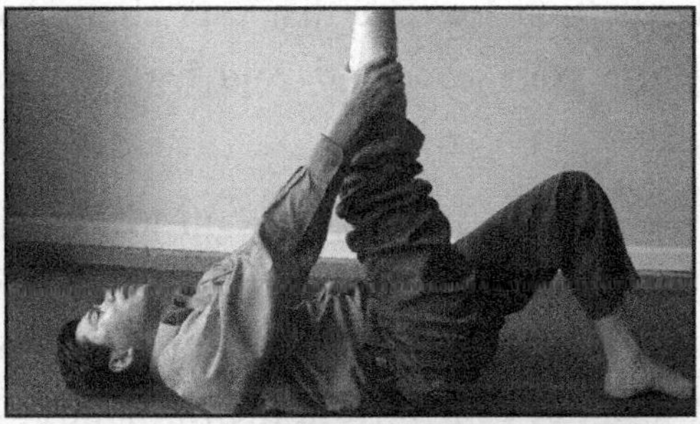

Lie straight on the floor and bring your leg toward your chest while grabbing onto the ankle or the calf area to help stretch the hamstring.

Quadriceps Stretches: Great for lower back pain and knee problems.

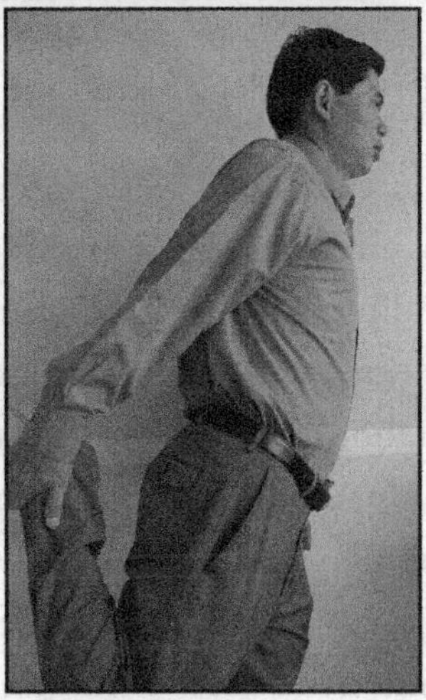

Grab your ankle or shin to stretch the quadriceps. Hold for forty to sixty seconds for a great stretch.

AEROBIC EXERCISE

Aerobic exercises require you to move very fast so your heart rate increases to 140 pulses per minute. These types of exercise include step aerobics, Tae Bo, running, and swimming. Aerobic exercise can be intense for people with joint problems or who have experienced head injuries because the rapid movement can cause dizziness. Aerobic exercise is more suitable for those who have a lot of energy and are fit and healthy. However, swimming is one aerobic exercise that seems to suit people of all ages with many different conditions. Swimming is great for patients with arthritis, for children, and for senior citizens. It is actually the only exercise that uses almost every part of your body, from your arms and your legs to your head and your lungs.

Aerobic exercises are great for weight loss when combined with weight training. However, the goal of all exercise is never to overwork your body because if your body becomes too stressed, you will not benefit from the workout.

ANAEROBIC EXERCISE

Anaerobic exercise is very intense because it causes your body to go into anaerobic metabolism, such as for example in bodybuilding. Lifting large amounts of weight and doing many repetitions will increase muscle mass which leads to increased metabolism by increasing the fat burning hormones. The goal of anaerobic exercise is to build more muscle fibers. Muscle is great for tonicity, but too much may not be good for those who just want to be toned. So these exercises are solely for bodybuilders, or those who want to gain some muscle mass and then go back to aerobic exercises as their daily routine.

Anaerobic exercise is where our body actually uses up all the glycogen stored in the body, which is why bodybuilders hardly have any fat on them. Remember, glycogen is a form of stored sugar processed in the liver when excess sugar is floating around in the bloodstream. Thus, if our body has a lot of stored fat cells or a person is diabetic, weightlifting is a great exercise not only to reduce fat but also to reduce blood sugar because our body uses up the sugar in the form of the energy needed to perform the anaerobic type of exercise.

For most people, however, current studies show that vigorous exercise is not healthy, especially for those with chronic conditions. It is recommended that people only increase their heart rates about 60 percent during a workout and aerobic exercise.

Of course, before you go out and start lifting 200 lbs of weight, have your health evaluated by your doctor. Then start off slow. Begin with 5-10 lbs weights, and do three sets of ten repetitions; then each week, increase the weight in accordance with your body's tolerance level. I would recommend working with an exercise trainer first to get a good idea of what is appropriate for your body; then later, you can go out and do it by yourself.

Persistence is the key in everything. Your body will begin to lose weight if you are persistent for more than thirty days. And as the weight begins to come off, make sure your body is well nourished to accommodate the constant demand made upon it by exercise. By eating healthy food rich in vitamins and minerals, you will lose weight faster and build more lean muscle.

Chapter 7

EXERCISE RECOMMENDATIONS

When exercising, it is key not to overwork your body. You actually do more damage than provide benefits to your body when you overwork it. According to a New York Medical Center study, men who exercise long and vigorously enough to break a sweat five to seven days a week have an increased chance of Atrial Fibulation (AF). AF can progress to heart failure and stroke. When we overwork the body, it causes our adrenal gland to become overstressed. Our natural fight-flight instinct actually kicks in everytime we exercise; we activate the adrenal glands, which puts stress on them, causing a release of the hormone called cortisol, which actually turns off the fat burning hormones.

The best way to exercise is to pay attention to how your body feels—remember it gives you pain and other signs of what it needs. That's why I recommend you find a chiropractor to serve as your fitness coach. You should always be evaluated by a chiropractor before you begin to workout so you can make sure your spine is in alignment and your body will be able to withstand the demands of exercise. Once a chiropractor makes certain that your bones and muscles are in alignment, you can workout with a fitness trainer to accomplish your exercise goals without pain and discomfort.

I often hear from patients, "I workout even though I am in pain." Well, if you are in pain, something is not structurally correct and the body is giving you a sign to check out what is wrong.

When it comes to exercise, you want an activity you can perform daily without feeling like you have to force yourself to do it. Exercise should be productive and fun. If you don't think it is fun, pick an activity that is fun. For example, when I am in the bathroom brushing my teeth, I will do twenty-five reps of squatting while brushing my teeth. After I finish brushing my teeth, I will do a triceps press on the tub for another twenty-five reps. I follow that with one hundred alternating kicks in the air, and I finish it off with twenty push-ups. Of course, sometimes I alternate or vary it, but that is my basic morning routine before I get dressed for the day. The rest of the day I choose to do different exercise activities ranging from walking or jogging for two miles to gardening or house cleaning.

Exercise should be fun and fulfilling. To start your body off properly, start slowly and increase with intensity. You don't have to start with a one- or two-hour or all day workout. As long as you are moving, your body is using the energy. You are burning fat so when you then eat healthy foods, your body can use the nutrients to build stronger cells.

I usually exercise to stay toned. To get tonicity is to build more muscle mass, which involves high intensity and short durations. The body recognizes that muscle tonicity equates to youthfulness. Dr. Stephen Cherniske states that "muscle mass sends a longevity signal to the brain." That is why people with muscle tonicity tend to look a lot younger and to have more energy. So exercise not only to lose weight, but to look young, build muscle tonicity, release toxins from your body, and ultimately, have a long, healthy, and pain-free life.

My favorite exercise of all is gardening, but we all have different hobbies we enjoy. To get the most out of your exercise investment, I recommend a thirty minute activity accompanied by the following:

- Stretch before and after each workout.
- Drink 8 oz. of water before your workout, 8 oz. throughout the workout, and then another 8 oz. after the workout. This will keep your body hydrated throughout the entire workout.
- Always eat a large amount of vegetables and protein with no carbohydrates for breakfast before you workout in the morning. A lot of people skip breakfast before they go to workout. If you eat and workout, you tend to burn more calories.
- Wear comfortable shoes and clothing.
- Exercise with the reason to release toxins so your body can function at its optimal level. Weight loss, beauty, and youthfulness will then just come naturally.
- Know your normal BMI and set a target to reach that goal.
- Monitor your heart rate, and make sure not to get it up too high.

- Have a chiropractor as your fitness coach.

Exercising and keeping those tips in mind will allow you to keep your body in optimal health. That's why exercise is the second investment necessary to achieve a healthy life.

Section 3

TOXINS

These residents are frightened. They woke up one day and found out that they are living in a toxic waste dump. They have learned that they had been drinking water that can cause cancer. They are rightfully scared for their well-being and for the well-being of their children.

– Gary Kendall

Chapter 8

WHAT ARE TOXINS?

In Section Two, I briefly talked about toxins and the body's system of eliminating toxins. Toxins are everywhere in our lives. We are constantly bombarded by toxic chemicals in our food, water, and air. Toxins are poisonous chemicals that need to be eliminated from the body to prevent harm because if they stay in our bodies they can accumulate until they overwhelm our immune systems. Furthermore, toxins limit our ability to lose weight, to get a good night's sleep, and to think clearly; they also cause a host of illnesses such as leaky gut syndrome, asthma, and cancer.

In this chapter, I will address four kinds of toxins:

1. Chemical
2. Environmental
3. Radiation and Electromagnetic
4. Emotional

All of these toxins cause havoc to our immune system and can lead to chronic illnesses such as cancer. Our children are especially vulnerable to deadly toxins because their bodies are still growing and their immune systems are still developing. According to a report in the medical journal *Lancet*, "Fetal and early childhood exposures to hundreds of chemical contaminants are causing a silent pandemic of brain disorders."

Let's look at where these toxins are originating, and how we can protect our loved ones and ourselves from them so we can reduce the level of toxins accumulating in our bodies.

1. CHEMICAL TOXINS

Chemical toxins are found everywhere in our daily lives. So far, over 10,000 known chemicals are used daily in every facet of our lives. Some of the most common ones we are exposed to daily are:

- Food
- Water
- Air
- Vaccines
- Drugs and Medication
- Heavy Metals
- Our Homes
- Cosmetics
- Clothing

Let's take a closer look at each one.

Food

The most consumed and most advertised product containing toxins is food. We are a society that loves to eat. We love to super-size our meals and eat to the point where we can no longer take one more bite. Furthermore, the foods we eat contain food additives to make us addicted to a food, which drives us to eat more and more of that same food.

Food additives such as MSG are known to cause damage to our body, especially to the brain. Do you ever feel tired or sleepy or have you had headaches after eating a meal rich in MSG? That is because MSG overexcites our brain cells to the point that they die.

Worst of all is deep fried food because the unhealthy oil used is toxic. Vegetable oils, corn oil, and canola oil are not good for frying because they are unstable. High heat causes their molecular bonds to break, which damages our body because hydrogenated or trans fat can block our body's ability to absorb and use the essential fats. Instead, the fat clogs the artery and creates free radicals in the body which can lead to cancer.

How about refined carbohydrates? A lot has been discussed on this topic, but what does it mean and how is it affecting our body? Refined carbohydrates are foods that have had their vitamins, minerals, and other nutrients removed while being processed; examples are white flour, candies, soda pop, cakes, and cookies. These foods have no nutritious value and are loaded with toxins. For example, the sugar in the soda pop or in cookies is more sugar than the body needs to process into energy, so the body stores the excess sugars as fat. The excess sugar stops the fat burning hormones from using the fat as energy.

Other chemical toxins found in our foods come from added chemicals like pesticides, additives, antibiotics, and hormones. These toxic chemicals are the leading cause of cancer. Research has linked asthma, cancer, and neurodevelopmental disorder to chemical exposures. Chemicals such as growth hormones and antibiotics are frequently used in chickens, pigs, and cows to speed up the growth process so they can be slaughtered and sold faster at the market. Pesticides are used regularly to grow the fruits and vegetables to prevent bugs from eating them. Pesticides are also found in the home in the form of insect killer sprays. Chronic exposure to pesticides can lead to nerve damage, skin disorders, and cancer.

Water

Water is the life force and the miraculous healer of our bodies since 70-80 percent of the body is made up of water. It acts as the body's electrolyte that energizes the body, removes toxins, and cleanses. We consume water daily.

But the tap water in our homes is also depleting our health because of all the chlorine and other toxic chemicals placed in it. Some toxic chemicals found in water include industrial solvents, weed killers, refrigerants, gasoline, cleaning products, a rocket fuel component called percolate, and prescription drugs like birth control pills and anti-depressants. Another chemical is chlorine, which is a dangerous free radical that contributes to cancer and aging, yet it is added regularly to tap water. Clean, chemical-free water is hard to find.

According to a recent report from scientificamerican.com, over 200 unregulated chemicals were found in the tap waters of forty-five states. In the United States, the Environmental Protection Agency (EPA) only has regulation over 114 of those chemicals. The Ralph Nader Study Group, after reviewing over 10,000 documents, concluded that "U.S. drinking water contains more than 2,100 toxic chemicals that can cause cancer." And the Federal Council on Environmental Quality reported that more than two-thirds of cancers may be attributed to low level toxins; even a small amount of toxin exposure can cause cancer. However, our body is constantly bombarded with all kinds of toxic chemicals.

Recommendations: If you are living close to an artesian well, I would highly recommend taking advantage of it. Here in Lynnwood, Washington, we have an artesian well that is tested monthly by the Alderwoods Water and Wastewater District for safety. Its water tastes great, especially when you get it right off the well. It is cold and fresh. If you are not fortunate enough to have an artesian well in your area, buy bottled spring water or mineral water. Another solution is to buy a water filter to filter out some of the chemicals found in the tap water. Lastly, boil the tap water if you have to drink it.

Air

Air is another essential need of our bodies; air is to the human body what gas is to the car. But our air is contaminated with all sorts of chemical toxins, and most of those toxins are found in our homes. Some of the chemicals found in the air are chlorine, fluorine, formaldehyde, pesticides, solvents from diesel and diesel exhaust products, and vanadium, a by-product of burning petroleum and petroleum products.

Even knowing how to breathe properly, as I discussed in Chapter 5, doesn't guarantee optimal health since our air is polluted. According to EPA reports in 1985, the air in our home is three times more toxic than the air outdoors. The toxic chemicals in our homes include mold, carpeting, paints, and cleaning products. Poor ventilation in our homes is a major contributing factor that allows chemical toxins to accumulate in the air and ultimately in our bodies.

Recommendations: Ventilate the house as much as possible. Open all the windows and doors when it is sunny and warm, especially in the morning to get the freshest oxygen without the pollution of car exhaust. Avoid using aerosol sprays.

Finally, having plants in the home will help to clean polluted air. They absorb toxic fumes in the air including benzene, formaldehyde, and trichloroethylene, and they produce fresh oxygen out of the carbon dioxide in the air. A NASA study on the best plants to filter a space station's air recommended the following plants:

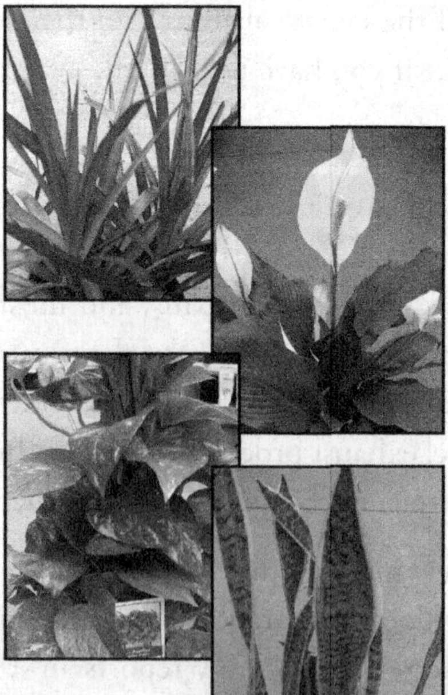

- Spider Plants: reduce air pollution
- Peaceful Lily: a great absorbent of benzene, formaldehyde, and other toxic fumes
- Heartleaf Philodendron: superb at cleaning and purifying the air
- Elephant Ear Philodendron: removes toxic air
- Red Edge Dracaena: great for filtering formaldehyde
- Janet Craig Dracaena:

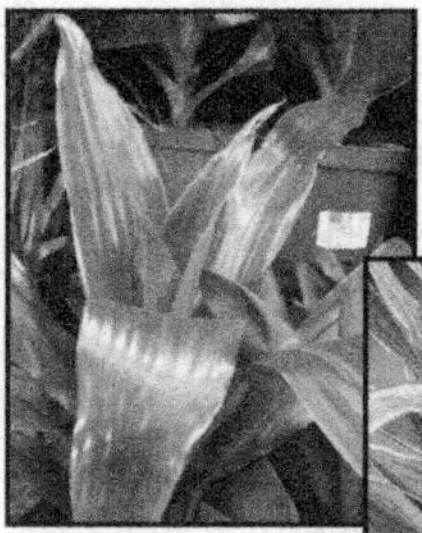

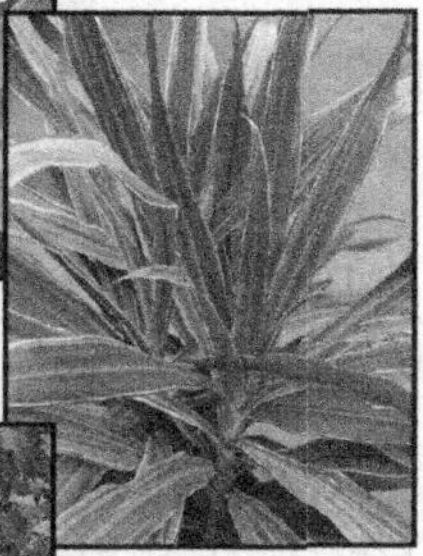

great for filtering formaldehyde and xylene

- Warneck Dracaena: great for filtering formaldehyde and xylene
- Weeping Fig: very effective as an indoor air filter

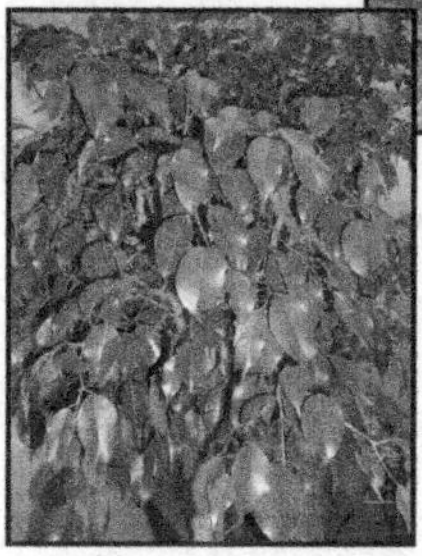

Vaccines

This topic is a very sensitive and controversial one. The choice to vaccinate your child should be up to each individual parent. Many parents whose children have been greatly affected by vaccines feel that having their child vaccinated was the cause of their son or daughter's health problems. For example, earlier I mentioned Jenny McCarthy, whose son was diagnosed with autism. He had no signs of autism until after he was given his vaccination shots. Although pediatricians claim there are no studies showing a relationship between vaccinations and autism, many parents of autistic children are convinced by ample evidence and research that vaccinations are responsible for their children's health problems.

Do vaccines even really help to save lives? According to U.S. Government data, the drop in deaths from the measles is the result in the improvement of living standards including better hygiene, water purification, and efficient sewage systems, not vaccines. And according to WHO, the chance of contracting measles is fourteen times greater if you are vaccinated against the disease. Furthermore, the death rate caused by measles in Massachusetts from 1860-1970 dropped prior to the introduction of measles vaccines in 1963 as an improvement in living standards.

A November 22, 1997 article published in the *Journal of Science*, called "The Dark Side of Immunization," concluded, after reviewing reports from several countries, that children who are vaccinated have a higher incidence of behavioral problems, asthma, diabetes, and a lower IQ than children who are not vaccinated. Thus, not only did the vaccines not protect our children from the disease, but vaccination caused more harm to their innocent lives.

Another study found that the doctors and scientists on the staff of the National Institute of Health during the 1950s were well aware that the SALK (polio) vaccine was "ineffective and deadly," yet they went ahead with letting the vaccine be given to America's children.

According to Dr. Baillie-Hamilton, "Ever since mass vaccination of infants began in the 20th Century reports of serious brain, cardiovascular, metabolic and other injuries started filling pages of medical journals." Dr. Baillie-Hamilton went on to say "children are at a higher risk than adults because their immune systems of detoxification are still developing which causes damage by the chemicals in the vaccines leading to autism."

Some of the reported side-effects experienced by children as the result of vaccines are:

- Sudden Infant Death
- Brain Damage
- MS
- Autism
- ADHD
- Dyslexia
- Eczema
- Asthma
- Diabetes
- Autoimmune Problems
- Seizures

As you can see, the listed sides effects are all issues we are currently seeing children repeatedly diagnosed with today. Asthma, eczema, diabetes, and autism have become common household conditions now. Almost every child now has a case of eczema. You don't need a doctor's degree to know what eczema is since it is so well known. It was not that common, however, fifty years ago when these conditions were almost unheard of. How about autism? Today, 1 in every 110 children is diagnosed with autism—an alarming rate.

How about diabetes? This condition is so life threatening to young children, and it is now an epidemic. This condition used to be an adult onset, but for the last two decades, we have seen it rise in young children. According to the Centers for Disease Control (CDC), in 2001, 3.5 million children under the age of twenty developed diabetes. By 2002, that number had jumped to 5.5 million—those results are staggering!

And what about ADHD? According to the CDC, 4.5 million children were diagnosed with ADHD in 2006 alone! And how do we treat these children? With more medication, which just means more drugs with more side effects. WOW!

Could vaccines be the cause of these increased health issues? Vaccines definitely introduce toxins into our bodies in the form of chemicals and animal tissues. Below are the toxic ingredients included in some of the most frequently used vaccines:

Polio Vaccine

- Neomycin: antibiotics used to treat infections; side-effects include allergies, bloody stools, seizures, muscle twitching, dizziness, hearing loss, and stomach cramps
- Streptomycin Sorbitol: antibiotics; side-effects include nausea, vomiting, fever, rash, and paresthesia of the face
- African Green Monkey Kidney cells: foreign object to the body; known to cause cancer. Read more at http://www.sv40foundation.org/Mission.html
- Calf Serum (blood from a three-month old cow): another species' blood entering our body to which we normally would never be exposed and which makes our body react negatively against because it is a foreign object.

Measles, Mumps, and Rubella Vaccines

- Rubella live virus
- Neomycin
- Chick embryonic fluid from eggs
- Human Diploids: cells from aborted fetus tissue

Diphtheria, Pertussis, and Tetanus Vaccines

- Formaldehyde: a known carcinogen
- Thermisal: a derivative of mercury
- Aluminum phosphate: solvents used as preservatives in place of mercury; toxic to the brain, liver, thyroid, and kidneys; linked to Alzheimer's disease
- Ammonium sulfate: also used as a preservative to replace mercury
- Washed sheep red blood cells: foreign tissue entering the body, causing the body to increase antibody production to fight it
- Glycerol: another preservative component; side-effects include possible skin disorders
- Sodium chloride: salt
- Pig pancreatic hydrolysate casein: foreign species tissue entering the human body that otherwise would never occur

As you can clearly see, these ingredients are chemicals and foreign animal tissues injected into our bodies. The first thing our body does when these vaccines are introduced is to respond by increasing the immune system's defense mechanisms. However, if our immune system is already weak or is not working, vaccines just compound the situation, causing the body to become sick and result in many health conditions.

As I said at the beginning of this discussion, vaccination is a very sensitive topic, so it is up to parents to make decisions for their individual children's health. I highly recommend doing all the research first. It is so easy now to obtain information thanks to the technology we have available.

Recommendations: Read and research before you make a decision whether or not to vaccinate your children. Some great sources are on the Internet, but Neil Z. Miller's book *Vaccines: Are They Really Safe and Effective?* would be a great place to start.

If you decide to vaccinate after you have read all the research, then make sure your child is well hydrated and is eating nutritiously. Also make sure your child gets plenty of sleep so the body can combat any fever that may follow the vaccination.

Drugs and Medication

A lot of Americans have been prescribed drugs and medication to help improve certain symptoms without a full understanding of the side-effects involved with their use. Because the body is an incredible machine that can withstand pretty much anything, we can swallow the strongest dose of medication or the maximum amount of alcohol, and the body will do its best to keep us alive by applying its detoxification mechanism system. Similarly, when we take medication, the medication must go through the filtering system of the liver and kidneys before it goes into the bloodstream and then to the organs, primarily the brain. Continued daily intake of over-the-counter (OTC) medication will, over time, overwhelm the liver.

OTC medications are widely used by Americans for pain. Most Americans think these constantly advertised medications are safe for daily use, but they are not. They are intended for temporary use only; use for prolonged periods will cause harmful damage to the body. Thousands of people die annually from constant use of OTC's, and hundreds of thousands suffer from incurable liver and kidney diseases.

Over 200 products containing acetaminophen are sold in the United States. For example, Tylenol is a great product to relieve temporary pain and to reduce fever. However, if you take one tablet everyday for one year, the liver will be compromised. How about Ibuprofen? Again, it is great for temporary use, but 1,000 pills over a lifetime can result in kidney damage. Aspirin is very popular and highly recommended by family doctors as a means of preventing heart disease, but its side-effects can include ulcers. Just read the labels on the medications you take and you'll see what are the side-effects.

According to the *Journal of the American Medical Association*, more than 100,000 people die each year from toxic reactions to prescription and OTC drugs. And patients who use OTC's as pain medications are more prone to developing chronic pain syndromes. Furthermore, Dr. Richard Besser of the CDC estimated that the number of unnecessary antibiotics prescribed annually for viral infections is 20 million.

Remember the sad news of Michael Jackson's tragic death in June 2009 from a prescription drug overdose? He was such a talented, kind, and loving artist, yet his body could no longer convert the toxic chemicals in his body. And let's not forget Elvis Presley, the "King of Rock and Roll." His addiction to pain medication caused him to die of a heart attack at age forty-two.

Recommendations: If you have ongoing pain that lasts for longer than a week and you have been on pain medications and yet are not experiencing relief, then go back to your family doctor and let him or her know you are still in pain. Also, find a local chiropractor and get a second opinion in regards to your pain. Working with both a chiropractor and your family doctor will greatly benefit your overall health. Remember, pain medication is designed to be a temporary solution, not ongoing or for a prolonged time period. Prolonged use has the danger of creating addiction, which is being seen far too often these days in patients who prolong pain medication without following up with their doctors.

Heavy Metals

We have heard about the dangers mercury can have on our health. But where does mercury come from and how does it enter the body? What other forms of heavy metals are there? How do they cause a health risk to the body? And what can we do to eliminate these heavy metal toxins from our bodies?

Mercury can be found in many fishes as well as in vaccines and dental fillings. Exposure to high doses of mercury can lead to permanent damage to the nervous system and kidneys.

Lead is another heavy metal that was commonly used in household paint until the U.S. Government banned it in 1977 from fear that children might ingest lead-based paint chips. Many older homes painted prior to that date still contain layers of such paint. Lead toxicity is dangerous to children under six years of age because it can cause damage to the nervous system, growth retardation, kidney damage, and delayed developmental skills. Lead may also be found in hazardous concentrations in food, water, and air.

Aluminum is widely used and can be found in a variety of products from vaccines to deodorants, and aluminum foils, pots, and pants. Because of its versatile use, aluminum has become a widely-used heavy metal, yet prolonged exposure to it can seriously affect our health. Aluminum can cause osteopenia because it competes with calcium for the body's receptors. High doses of aluminum can cause neurotoxicity and breast cancer.

Recommendations: The best way to eliminate toxic metals is to avoid them completely. Of course, that's not completely possible, but limit your exposure to them as much as possible. Read the labels of the products you put in and on your body. Eat healthy foods to strengthen your immune system's functions so they can combat these toxins. Drink plenty of purified water. And most importantly, exercise your body and mind.

Our Homes

Our home is our pride and joy. We work hard to buy a home for our families. Home is our sacred possession. Unfortunately, our home can be a hidden toxic burial ground for our family, filled with toxins from the carpet to the furniture, and from the paint on the walls to the cabinets.

Have you ever walked into a brand new finished home? Remember that new smell? No wonder we are so sick. The fumes in a house are toxic to breathe. Carpets are a health hazard because of the fibers, the fumes (arsenical pesticides, benzene, formaldehyde, toluene, acetone, plus many more), and the glue. Also, many carpet installers say they cannot buy life insurance because insurance companies know that the job makes them prone to lung cancer.

Dry wall is another toxic part of our homes. Dry wall contains toxic chemicals like formaldehyde and other toxic fumes. Do you remember the story of the dry wall made in China that contained toxic fumes? The fumes made so many people sick that they could no longer live in their home.

Furniture, especially new furniture, is also toxic because it contains formaldehyde.

We literally intoxicate our bodies with fumes coming from all directions in our homes. In fact, I remember that when my family moved into our new home, we were all sick for a week; it was because we were breathing in all the toxic fumes.

Recommendations: It is always best to have lots of plants to absorb the fumes as much as possible. And on a nice sunny day, vent your home as much as possible. I vent our home throughout the year. In the summer, I leave all the windows and even the door open. Venting in the morning is good feng shui because it brings good energy into the home, and in the morning, you get the freshest oxygen before all the cars and other pollutions of the day take place, filling the air with toxic fumes.

Cosmetics

I know we women feel like we cannot live without our makeup or cleansing products. However, we can still make ourselves look beautiful while not exposing our bodies to toxic chemicals.

Many beauty supplies contain chemicals that are hazardous to our health. For example, lipstick may contain lead, silicone, and aniline (a cancer-causing agent). According to a study in Frankfurt, Germany by Okeo, out of 306 lipsticks tested, including 21 different brands and various shades, 121 received a failing grade and another 44 were graded as "unsatisfactory."

What goes on our skin gets absorbed into our bodies. If we read the labels to find out the ingredients in lipstick, makeup, and many similar items, most of the time they include a long list of words we can't even pronounce, right?

Here are some of the basic toxic ingredients found in shampoos, deodorants, foundations, and lotions:

- **Mercury**: found in eye makeup; phenyl mercuric acetate is a highly toxic chemical used as a preservative in eye makeup.
- **Formaldehyde**: found in almost all care products including skincare, hair care, deodorant, and nail polish; formaldehyde exposure can cause joint or chest pain, depression, headaches, fatigue, dizziness, immune dysfunction, and cancer.
- **Mineral oil**: found in lotions to prevent water loss from the skin; can cause clogging of the skin, prevent the skin from removing toxins, and promote acne.
- **1-Naphthol and 2-Naphthol**: used as dye intermediates; derived from coal tar.
- **Lanolin**: derived from sheep's wool; found in many cosmetic products which contain organophosphate pesticide and insecticides; can cause cancer, behavior disorder, and disruptions to development of the brain, endocrine system, and nervous system.
- **Hexamethylenetetramine**: another form of formaldehyde found in cosmetics and lotions; a cancer-causing agent.

- **Nitrosamines**: a carcinogenic component.
- **(PHB Esters)**: used as a preservative; can cause allergic reactions and skin rashes.
- **Petrolatum**: impurities found in petroleum jelly; a carcinogen, believed to cause cancer including breast cancer.
- **Propylene Glycol**: comes from petroleum; can cause respiratory and throat irritation, central nervous system depression, blood and kidney disorder, and skin rashes.

As you can see, all of these chemical compounds enter our bodies daily without us being aware of it. And most women will not leave the house without putting on makeup. Over time, these toxic chemicals accumulate in our body's organs. Research has shown that chemical irritants are the number one factor in causing cancer.

Recommendations: To combat these toxins 1) start looking for products that are more organic and more natural, 2) eat healthy foods and exercise to eliminate the toxins from the body, and 3) limit use of the product whenever possible.

Clothing

We all know how we love fashion. For women especially, second only perhaps to makeup, clothes make us look and feel great. But what kinds of toxins, unaware to us, are hidden in our clothes?

Some of the ingredients used to make clothes contain fumes such as formaldehyde, and synthetic pesticides. All of these chemicals are toxic and irritants to the body. Exposure to them can impair our immune system functions.

Recommendations: Wear 100 percent wool or cotton that is natural. Items that are not natural are not healthy and do not provide the air our body needs to breathe. More clothing companies today are carrying organic clothing that does not use pesticides or formaldehyde in the clothing. Jonano.com is a great place for non-toxic clothing for women and children. Another great online store is mygreenlipstick.com, a one-stop shop place. REI stores are also great places for organic clothing.

2. ENVIRONMENTAL TOXINS

Look around and see if you can identify some of the toxins surrounding you and your family every day. Most toxins are so unnoticeable that we go about our daily lives without thinking twice about the harmful impacts they have upon our bodies.

Our environment is very important. Every part of our body is sensitive to everything around us. So to have a healthy life we need to be surrounded by a healthy environment. That means limiting exposure to noise and chemicals from household cleaning and other home products.

Noise

We live in a culture where we love to blast our televisions and radios, and we have to shout at each other when we talk, just to hear one another. Have you been to a party where all you can hear is noise and nothing else? You actually have to raise your voice to communicate with the person next to you.

Noise is defined as undesired sounds. Noise can be classified into two categories: 1) occupational (work), and 2) environmental (noise in all other settings), such as home, school, and community. Environmental noise resulting from daytime traffic, listening to loud music, and watching loud television programs all have a profound effects on adults and children. According to Dr. Lorraine E. Maxwell, Ph.D., "chronic exposure to noise has been shown to be harmful to children of all ages." For example, noise causes an increase in high blood pressure and decreases children's cognitive abilities. A WHO study found that long-term exposure to excessive noise has been responsible for thousands of premature deaths due to heart disease across the world.

Occupational noise mostly affects adults. According to a 1998 study by the National Institute for Occupational Safety and Health (NIOSH), over 30 million Americans are exposed to hazardous noise. Research done by WHO shows that the occupations whose workers are most at risk for noise-induced hearing loss include those in manufacturing, transportation, mining, construction, agriculture, and the military. A 2004 research study by de Hollander et al. showed noise can cause such health issues as annoyance, hypertension, disturbance of psycho-social wellbeing, and psychiatric disorders.

<u>Recommendations</u>: It is always a great idea to be a role model to your children. In our family, when we turn on the radio, we turn it on just loud enough to hear the music. Because our son is very sensitive to all things, his environment has to be right or we will pay the price. We turn the volume of the TV and radio only between volumes 6-8. Volume 8 is the loudest we will choose, and that is only when the car is moving.

Another tip is to shield your home from traffic, airplane,

and construction noise. If you can't move away or avoid the noise, have lots of plants inside the home to shield some of the noise and other toxins as well. Lastly, avoid areas or places that are noisy.

Plastic

Today, technology has made our lives so convenient, from communication to foods to household products. Plastic has become a means of living. Everywhere we look, we see a list of products that are made from plastic, from cooking utensils to food containers and water bottles, from groceries bags and garbage bags to baby bottles, baby pacifiers, and baby toys. Although, plastic bags have made our life more convenient, our planet and our own bodies are suffering from their hidden dangers. Our oceans especially are so polluted with plastic products, including water bottle containers, plastic grocery bags, and plastic soda pop holders that the lives of sea creatures are being threatened by their homes becoming less inhabitable for them. As for our human bodies, plastic containers contain such chemicals as Bisphenol A (BPA) and Phthalates, which have been found to cause disruptions in the endocrine system, brain disorder, and behavior disorder; they also trigger early puberty and breast development which are precursors to cancer.

3. RADIATION AND ELECTROMAGNETIC TOXINS

We are very fortunate to live in an era when man-made devices have made our lives much easier and more efficient. However, that efficiency comes with a price. To understand the consequences that modern technologies have on our bodies, we must first understand what they are.

Let's look at technologies we use daily in our homes. Look around and see how many devices you can identify. Imagine what each one of them is doing to your body. How has each one of these devices impacted your family's health? Let's just address a few popular items in the house such as the microwave, cell phone, and computer.

The Microwave

What a great invention! The microwave has saved millions of people time preparing and heating their meals. It speeds up time spent cooking by tenfold. It's so convenient for our busy lives. Some of us cannot live without a microwave because we are so dependent upon it.

How exactly does a microwave work and what does it do to our food?

A microwave works by dielectric heating, which means that microwave radiation heats the water molecules and other polarized molecules within the food. So when food is heated in the microwave, the water molecules in the food change their molecular compound, which in turn causes toxicity to our bodies since the food is no longer in its natural molecular state where our body can easily digest it. That is why microwaved food is harmful to our bodies. Recent research has shown that microwaved foods can cause cancer, and Dr. Hans Hertel, who performed extensive research into the dangers of microwaves, concluded that eating microwave cooked food caused increased levels of leukocytes in the body, which are an indication of cell damage.

A Russian investigation into the possible harmful effects of microwaves concluded that "carcinogens were formed in virtually all foods tested. No test food was subject to more microwaving than necessary to accomplish the purpose, i.e., cooking, thawing, or heating to insure sanitary ingestion."

Here is a list of results from the Russian Investigation study as published by the Atlantis Raising Educational Center in Portland, Oregon:

- Microwaving prepared meats sufficiently to insure sanitary ingestion caused formation of d-Nitrosodienthanolamines, a well-known carcinogen.
- Microwaving milk and cereal grains converted some of their amino acids into carcinogens.
- Thawing frozen fruits converted their glycosides and glucosides containing fractions into carcinogenic substances.
- Extremely short exposure of raw, cooked, or frozen vegetables converted their plant alkaloids into carcinogens.
- Carcinogenic free radicals were formed in microwaved plants, especially root vegetables, and decreased the plants' nutritional values.

Russian researchers also reported a marked acceleration of structural degradation leading to a decreased food value of 60 to 90 percent in all foods tested. Among the changes observed were:

- Decreased bioavailability of vitamin B complex, vitamin C, vitamin E, essential minerals and lipotropics factors in all foods tested.
- Various kinds of damage to many plant substances, such

as alkaloids, glucosides, galactosides, and nitrilosides.

- The degradation of nucleo-proteins in meats.

Cell Phones

How convenient is it to be able to talk to your loved one wherever and whenever? How about when you want your little girl to call you to let you know where she is at and what she is doing? I truly love having my cell phone around. I feel stranded without it, and I am sure most Americans feel the same way.

However, cell phones are now considered so dangerous that several states have made it illegal to talk on your cell phone (or text) while driving because too many lives have been lost as a result of driver distraction.

Besides people using their cell phones foolishly while driving, how else are cell phones creating a risk to our family's health? They can be dangerous primarily to children's brains—their brains are developing and filled with fluids, so when a cell phone is put near their ears, then just as a microwave heats up water molecules, the cell phone radiates children's brain cells. Over time, the result can be children developing brain tumors. According to Dr. Davra Davis, children are more vulnerable to brain tumors and hearing problems than adults because cell phone radiation penetrated deeper into the children's brains.

Adults are also at risk for brain tumors. In October 2009, after a $30 million study into cell phones and their relation to brain tumors, WHO reported that there is "a significantly increased risk" of some brain tumors "related to use of mobile phones for a period of ten years or more."

Computers

What a great invention is the computer. How can we function in today's high-tech society without this wonderful tool? It allows us to communicate with loved ones around the globe, to see and talk to them online, to store information, and to play games. How wonderful is that? Can you ask for anything more than this great machine?

Unfortunately, even this great device comes with a price. Computers emit electromagnetic fields (EMF) that are similar to those of cell phones. The electromagnetic field is made up of charged particles that move in motion, and when our bodies are exposed to that field, the particles enter our bodies, causing damage to our DNA, which ultimately can lead to headaches, insomnia, premature aging, leukemia in children, and brain cancer.

4. EMOTIONAL TOXINS

Our emotions are not toxic chemicals from outside our bodies, but they do cause our body stress, which then puts our body out of balance. Psychologist Karol Truman has studied the effects that different emotions have upon our body's health. In her book, *Feelings Buried Alive Never Die…*, she gives numerous examples, including how cancer results from self-destructive emotions, and how shoulder pain may result from family or financial issues. Low back pain may result from feeling unsupported financially or being unsupported in a relationship.

Obviously, we have all experienced emotions. But how we deal with our pain and suffering varies among individuals. Losing family members due to sickness, accident, and trauma may affect us in one way while relationship losses from break-ups and divorce may create different emotional responses such as anger co-mixed with grief. Whether you are mad at someone or someone is mad at you and making you sad, the emotions are buried somewhere inside your body, and those feelings can lead to toxic chemicals that then trigger the start of diseases.

Take, for example, depression. I had a male patient in his early twenties who came into my office in a wheelchair after he slipped and fell down the stairs in his house. He was left unable to move his legs or wiggle his toes. He was so depressed that he would not look at anyone and wanted nothing to do with anybody. He went about his daily life with his head constantly down. He felt so hopeless; I remember how his face was so dark and sad. His first couple of chiropractic treatments felt hopeless, but during his third treatment, when I adjusted his sacrum, it let out a loud pop. When he got off the table, I could see a glimmer of hope from him. As each treatment progressed, he was able to move his toes and gradually raise his leg off the table. By his seventh visit, he walked in with a crutch, and during his next visit, he had left his crutches at home. The joy on his face showed he was no longer feeling depressed and that chiropractic care had helped him regain the ability to walk.

Why is it important to understand emotional toxicity? In order for our body to heal itself completely, we need to address our emotional issues. Otherwise, painful and toxic emotions will linger and come back to attack us later in life in the form of diseases.

Once we are able to recognize emotional toxicity, we are able to release and let go of the past and move forward with love, joy, and health. Our life will have a different perspective for us. Thus, releasing the emotions we buried for years can be rejuvenating to our overall health.

An example of emotional toxicity in my own life resulted from when I was a little girl living in Cambodia during the Khmer Rouge regime. One day I was worried about my older sister, who claimed she was sick that morning, so I did not want to go to work in the rice fields but to stay behind and take care of her. But I was ordered to go to work. When I refused, the team leader and two other girls tried to drag me out of the boarding school. When I resisted, they kicked me and pulled my hair until I could no longer fend for myself. The team leader beat me until I was unconscious and believed to be dead. Then they just left me there in the room. I have no idea how long I remained unconscious, but it must have been more than eight hours. When I woke up, I was sweating, thirsty, and hungry. When I looked around, I saw my sister and the other girls in the group lining up for their dinner of sweet potatoes mixed with white rice. I remember my stomach grumbling, but I dared not make any noise. As I watched them eat their small portion of dinner, I cried myself back to sleep. I believe I was about six years old when this happened, but the emotion stayed buried inside of me for many years. Even after the bruises had long healed and I came to the United States, I would relive the event in my memory and my body would react with sick feelings. During my college years, I would find myself crying without reason while I was driving. When I came across Karol Truman's book *Feelings Buried Alive Never Die…* I began to understand the toxic emotions I was holding onto. Then I started to take meditation more seriously and began practicing it daily. I also began to stay away from people who were negative about everything and instead surrounded myself with positive people.

We all go through toxic emotions at different points in our lives. Those emotions could result from a divorce, someone betraying you, the death of a loved one, anger, guilt, jealousy, or loneliness. Remember Lorena Bobbitt? The emotional rage she experienced from her husband's abuse led her to do the unthinkable—cut off her husband's penis while he was sleeping. That just shows how our emotions can drives us to do things we would never contemplate if we were behaving rationally.

Our emotions affect our health and ultimately how we live. If our body is harboring toxic emotions, the results can manifest in our lives in areas least expected; these emotions will usually be aroused when we are under pressure, and besides not making us feel good, they could cause us to act in ways we later regret. Thus, by releasing these emotions we can move on with our lives and live a healthier life.

Ways to Heal Emotions

The best way to heal any emotional pain is to give it time. To heal truly difficult emotions, we need to look at the bigger perspective and consider all the joyful things life has to offer rather than just playing over and over in our heads the split moment that created the toxic emotion. Those who have severe emotional issues should, of course, seek professional help. Find a psychologist or psychiatrist who can help to get you back on track to healthy living.

I also recommend being around positive friends and people

who have a positive outlook on life. Also try practicing meditation; it can bring peace into our souls and take us to a more spiritual level. Meditation is the best way to keep our mind, body, and spirit feeling whole so we can let go of the unnecessary emotions inside of us. Exercise is also important to relieve toxic emotions; research studies have proven that exercise helps people be less depressed. Finally, find ways to make yourself laugh—watching comedy programs is great for helping us to forget our sadness.

EXERCISES

What toxic chemical products do you have in your home that you can do without?

What are three things that make you smile or feel happy?

What three plants would you truly enjoy having in your home that would eliminate the most toxins?

Chapter 9

DETOXIFICATION

As you can see, our body is under tremendous stress not just from the toxicity all around us, but also from eating non-nourishing foods, lack of exercise, and the daily demands we request our body to perform. No wonder our bodies seems to be low in energy and we look everywhere for a quick fix to boost our energy level in the form of caffeine products such as coffee, soda, or energy drinks like Red Bull. We go about our daily lives with these temporary energy boosts to get us through the day, and then we come home to an even more depleted life by staying up late, eating unhealthy foods, and not exercising. This cycle repeats itself day after day, month after month, and year after year. No wonder we are starting to see all sorts of health conditions on the rise, including diabetes, cancer, hypertension, and stroke. These illnesses are common household names now, and we have become accustomed to learning to live with them. But do you really have to live with chronic pain and debilitating disease, or can you do something about it?

The answer is clear. If our body is so bombarded by the overwhelming burden of toxins, non-nutritious foods, and lack of exercise, we need to turn this situation around. That means detoxifying our body of all the toxins in it. Detoxification is the third principle investment to achieving optimal health. But how do we make the investment?

Detoxification of our body is like taking your car to a mechanic to get an oil change every three thousand miles. Have you ever looked at how filthy the old oil is when it is changed? The same scenario happens to our blood after years of accumulating toxins from refined foods, alcohol, medication, and all the other toxins to which our bodies are exposed. When we detoxify our bodies, we are cleaning the blood system, and in turn, we are cleaning all the organ systems of the waste that has accumulated in them over the years. Or think of detoxification as being like spring-cleaning. Just as we set aside time in the spring to clean our homes to get rid of unwanted clothes, garbage, and dirt that has accumulated over the years, we need to make the same time commitment to our bodies. We need to set a time to clean our bodies, and the best time to do it is in the spring so we can get our bodies ready for a beautiful summer—not just so we can look great in a swimsuit, but because this time supports the spleen and liver meridian; if our spleen is not functioning at its optimal level, it's because its meridian points are blocked and preventing the harmonious flow of energy. For instance, since our spleen is responsible for the transportation and transformation of different substances in the body, a sluggish spleen function can lead to a decrease in our health. Individuals with spleen dysfunctions may experience symptoms like abdominal distention, diarrhea, flatulence, and a heavy sensation of the body. As for the liver meridian, a dysfunction of the liver can lead to such symptoms as skin rashes, sinus problems, migraines, PMS, and an inability to lose weight.

An annual spring-cleaning of our bodies should begin with fasting. Fasting allows the body to cleanse out all the toxic waste accumulated in our intestinal lining, our liver, and all the organs that normally could not be released due to the continual dump of waste into the body. When we fast, we give our bodies a break. We give our digestive tract the ability to clean itself from all that waste. Remember, 80 percent of our immune system is in the digestive tract, so if our digestive tract is blocked with toxins, then it decreases our immune system. To reverse this situation and increase our immune functions, we must have a healthy digestive tract. Once our digestive tract is healthy, we are better able to absorb the nutrients we eat and to combat foreign objects such as a virus from the common cold or flu. Detoxification is like keeping our home spotless for a couple of weeks.

Furthermore, spring-cleaning our body from toxins allows us to lose weight easily, sleep better, and think better. Our overall health is much improved because our body is able to absorb all the nutrients we eat and then use them to provide us with more energy. Because an unhealthy GI tract is not good for your overall health, even if we practice healthy eating and we exercise, without addressing this underlying issue, we will not lose weight or obtain optimal health.

RECOMMENDATIONS:

- Work with a chiropractor who specializes in detoxification. You can also try Dr. Brantley's three-day detoxification program at www.brantleycure.com or Dr. Paula Baillie-Hamilton's detoxification program as explained in her book *The Detox Diet.*
- Visit doctors or chiropractors who use the Brimhall Technique for body cleansing (see www.brimhall.com for more information).
- Get regular spinal care.
- Exercise regularly.
- Eat nutritious foods.
- Have plants in your home.
- Ventilate your home as often as possible.
- Buy an electric and magnetic field shield device.
- Visit www.electropolution.org to find cell phone and computer device protection.

Section 4

SPINAL HEALTH

Physicians of the highest rank—To pay whose fees would need a bank—Have pressed their science, art, and skill Into a dose of calomel. Whate'er the patient may complain Of head, or heart, or nerve, or brain, Of fever high, or parts that swell—The remedy is calomel. When Mr. A. or B. is sick, "Go for the doctor; and be quick." The Doctor comes with right good will, And ne'er forgets his calomel. He turns unto the patient's wife, And asks for the paper, spoon, and knife; "I think your husband will do well To take a dose of calomel." He then deals out the fatal grain, "This ma'am, will surely ease the pain, Once in three hours, at chime of bell, Give him a dose of calomel." The man grows worse quite fast indeed, A council's called. They ride with speed. They crowd around his bed, and tell The man to take more calomel. The man in death begins to groan, The fatal job for him is done. His falt'ring voice in death doth tell His friends to shun all calomel. Now, when I must yield up my breath, Pray let me die a natural death, And bid you all the long farewell Without the use of calomel..

– "Calomel", a mid-nineteenth-century song

Chapter 10

CHIROPRACTIC HISTORY

To understand chiropractic in relation to our spinal health and our overall wellbeing, we must first travel down the path of history to learn how chiropractic began. Then we'll explore the role of chiropractic in healthcare medicine today, and most importantly, why you should see a chiropractor.

Chiropractic began in 1895 when Dr. D.D. Palmer discovered that by adjusting the spine, he had cured the hearing loss of a janitor named Harvey Lillard. After his success with Lillard, Dr. Palmer treated another patient who had a heart condition; he found the patient had a subluxated vertebra in the spine, but with an adjustment, the problem was resolved. Following these successes, Dr. Palmer began to study anatomy, physiology and neurology and discovered that when the nervous system is blocked or experiences interference, disease can occur. This discovery was the answer to his burning question, "What is life?" and why out of two individuals who eat at the same table and work in the same environment, one may become sick while the other remains well. The doctor concluded that the nervous system determines the individual's quality of life. Any interference to the nervous system will diminish a person's health. Thus, after realizing the powerful effects of spinal adjustment, Dr. Palmer started to treat all his patients with his new discovery.

By 1896, Dr. Palmer, convinced of the power of these techniques for his patients' wellbeing and their potential to help millions more people in the future, asked the Reverend Samuel Weed to help him to come up with a name for this spectacular treatment. Prior to that, Samuel Weed had thought Dr. Palmer was a quack, until his daughter suffered a life-threatening ankle-sprain and went to see Dr. Palmer; with one adjustment, she felt so much better that she walked home holding her crutches. A year later, the reverend sought treatment for his sciatica, so Dr. Palmer made a barter arrangement with Rev. Weed to pay for his treatment; he asked the reverend to find a dignified Greek name for his new healing method. And you guessed it—chiropractic was the name Rev. Weed chose. In Greek, chiropractic means "done by hand." And that was the beginning of chiropractic.

Dr. Palmer was so successful at treating patients with all sorts of ailments that in 1897 he opened a chiropractic school. By 1908, chiropractic had spread like a virus to Great Britain, and by the early 1920s, it was being practiced in most countries on the seven continents.

Today, chiropractors can be found worldwide and chiropractic is widely accepted and respected, yet most Americans are still not fully aware of what chiropractic is, and they remain wary of seeing a chiropractor. The reasons for this caution and unfamiliarity stem back to the early 1900s when chiropractic was given a bad name by the medical community, led by the American Medical Association (AMA) and osteopaths.

In the early twentieth century, medical doctors wanted to be the only ones who could practice medicine so they strove to pass the Medical Practice Act, which would put anyone in jail who practiced medicine without a license, and chiropractors were not granted medical licenses. Thus, Dr. Palmer himself and several other chiropractors were put in jail. Chiropractors took enormous risks in those days to help their patients, especially because medical doctors would hire people to pose as patients, called "spotters" or "sneakers," to see what treatments were being given in chiropractic offices.

To counteract this situation and avoid being sued for practicing medicine without a license, chiropractors had patients sign a piece of paper that described all treatments in non-chiropractic terms so the document could be used in court to "offset any misstatement made by the sneakers." And when sneakers would testify in court with false statements, patients of arrested chiropractors would show up to testify to the benefits of their chiropractic treatments.

The quarrel of medical doctors and osteopaths against chiropractors continued into the mid-twentieth century. Allopathic journals of the time commonly included stories with such headlines as: "Chiropractor Indicted on Charge of Manslaughter," "Patient Dies in Chiropractor's Office," or "Neck-Twisted Patient Dies."

By 1963, the American Medical Association (AMA) established a Committee on Quackery whose main goal was to "contain and eliminate chiropractic." The editor of the AMA journal issued statements that any hospitals or medical doctors who work with chiropractors or practiced forms of chiropractic would lose their accreditation with the AMA. The result to this day is that few hospitals have chiropractors on staff.

In the years immediately following, the AMA published an exposé titled *At Your Own Risk* about the dangers of chiropractic. It then mailed out hundreds of copies of this book to every state medical society in the U.S., every national medical society worldwide, and to the 1,200 largest libraries in the U.S.

Chiropractors responded to these allegations with poise and substantial proof of chiropractic's value. Dr. Chester A. Wilk, one of the most respected chiropractors, responded with *Chiropractic Speaks Out*, a well-written book in which he compiled hard facts and scientific evidence to reply to the propaganda, bigotry, and ignorance of the medical profession.

Chiropractic continued to be treated as less authentic than other forms of medicine in 1965 when Medicare's reimbursement system was established. Even though chiropractors wanted to be included as providers covered by the plan, along with allopathic and osteopathic physicians under the system, they were left out. Upon chiropractors' requests to Congress, the Secretary of Health, Education, and Welfare investigated chiropractic to determine the merit of the request to be included as providers, but the request was denied because "the theory and practice are not based upon the body of basic knowledge related to health, disease, and health care that has been widely accepted by the scientific community." Chiropractors fought back by encouraging patients to write to their congressmen to ask that chiropractors be included in Medicare's reimbursement system. An estimated twelve million letters and telegrams poured into Congress, with people detailing how chiropractic had helped them and their families and requesting chiropractors be included as providers in Medicare's reimbursement system. The endless letters continued to pour into Congress' offices daily until finally in 1974, chiropractors became accepted providers according to Medicare.

Two years later, Dr. Chester Wilk and four other chiropractors filed a lawsuit against the AMA for violation of the Sherman Antitrust Act. The charge was that the AMA's purposes were primarily economic in an attempt to restrain competition by chiropractors. The court battle dragged on for over ten years until 1987 when the U. S. District Court for the Northern District of Illinois decided against organized medicine in the case of Wilk vs. AMA. An injunction then was issued permanently forbidding the AMA "from restricting, regulating or impeding" any of its members or any hospitals or other medical institutions from professionally associating with chiropractors. And the AMA was ordered by the court to publish the entire ruling in the *Journal of the American Medical Association* and the *American Medical News* to notify its members that they were now allowed without threat of losing their licenses to refer patients to, accept patients from, and to be associated with chiropractors. The AMA's attempt to appeal this decision was refused by the U.S. Supreme Court in 1994.

After the victories regarding Medicare and this lawsuit against the AMA, chiropractors were added to most health insurance, worker's compensation insurances, and the IRS allowed taxpayer deductions for chiropractic care as part of medical expense.

Although chiropractors have won the battle legally, becoming accepted by the general public is still a long uphill climb. Not until fairly recently (1991) did the chiropractic profession begin to receive small grants from the federal government to fund research, and even today, most patients will first go to a doctor for their aches and pains rather than seeing a chiropractor. Medical doctors still tend more often to refer patients with low back and neck pain to physical therapists or orthopedic surgeons rather than to chiropractors, and some medical doctors and patients still remain unaware of the practices and benefits of chiropractic. For example, I still have patients who upon their first visits tell me, "I heard chiropractors are dangerous. They can break your bones" or "My doctor told me to go see a physical therapist instead." But once the patients receive chiropractic treatment, they wish they had started sooner.

Following is a story from one of my patients about her preconceptions about chiropractic care and how experiencing chiropractic care firsthand changed that perception:

Initially, I was skeptical about chiropractic treatments because of friends and coworkers' experiences with chiropractors. I thought I would never have to encounter one until I sustained a whiplash injury from a car accident in 2007 and experienced chronic neck pain and persistent, throbbing, unbearable headaches. Hesitantly, by recommendation, I had no choice but to go to a chiropractor and met Dr. Jeudi. Not only was she very professional, but she was extremely personable and amiable. She cares about not only my injured body but my wellbeing. I have witnessed her holistic approach, and she goes out of her way for her patients' complete healing. She is exceptional and extraordinary, and I will be forever grateful! Now I'm a believer in chiropractic treatments; as a matter of fact, I recommend Dr. Jeudi to my family and friends." — **Alma Duran.**

Despite the public's lack of information about the value of chiropractic, research studies show that chiropractic is a safer and more effective course of treatment than conventional medicine, especially today when studies have shown that over 100,000 Americans die each year as the result of medical errors, estimated as more than the number who die from traffic accidents, or diseases such as diabetes, Alzheimer's, or pneumonia.

So why have we not yet seen wide acceptance of chiropractors? I believe the past damage done by the AMA and osteopaths still has its effects today. But perceptions are beginning to change. Chiropractors are now receiving privileges in hospital settings, and more medical doctors are referring their patients to chiropractors. And in Washington State, a survey showed that more than two-thirds of medical doctors agreed that, "chiropractic treatment is effective for some patients." The battle for patients to have the effective care they deserve is finally being won.

Chapter 11

CHIROPRACTIC PHILOSOPHY

The spinal column holds, we know, a most important place.
When normal, it is beauteous, a form of wondrous grace.
But when distorted, it becomes the seat of many ills,
Which are, frequently, mistreated with ineffective pills.
Adjust the subluxations till crooked spines grow straight.
Take off from nerves the pressure which induce (sic) an evil state.
Thus many ailments vanish and health appears for all
Who, wisely, on Dame Nature for real assistance call....
Away with drugs which poison and instruments that kill.
Let us use, in wisdom's way, of mental, manual skill.
The hands, by mind directed, can drive our ills away
And bring us advantageous health for which we all shall pray.

Chiropractic is founded on the tenets of philosophy, art and science. Chiropractic philosophy states that the patient's body has the power to heal itself, and the chiropractor just assists the body to free itself from restrictions. For that reason, many chiropractic offices have posters that contain such sayings as, "The Power that made the body heals the body" and "Innate

Intelligence knows."

Dr. Palmer understood the body's healing abilities. He stated, "Given the right environment and free of blockage, the innate power is free to flow." He knew that all of life's phenomena were activated by the impulse of the Innate Intelligence transmitted through the nervous system.

According to Dr. Palmer, "to heal a patient, a chiropractor just needs to correct the subluxated vertebra. By correcting the subluxated vertebra, the body's innate intelligent restores itself." Dr. Palmer went on to say "Chiropractors remove the obstacles to nature's healing processes."

Chiropractors have great respect for the human body because it is an amazing machine that has the intelligence to heal and replicate itself. Chiropractors believe that the body's innate intelligence knows from the time of inception that the brain and the spinal cord are the two most important organs of the body. That is why those organs are protected with hard shells: the skull in the head and twenty-four movable spinal vertebrae in the spine. Chiropractors understand that if the communication between the brain and the spinal cords are somehow blocked, optimal health is diminished, which can lead to a variety of chronic diseases if not treated. Furthermore, chiropractors also understand that doctors do not heal; only the patient's innate intelligence can heal his or her body, but chiropractors assist the body by detecting the obstacles blocking the flow of life and restoring the body to normal. Chiropractors are the mechanics of the human body, just as the auto-mechanic is for a car. Once the chiropractic removes the obstacles, the body returns to its natural homeostasis. The body desires nothing more than to be in a state of balance, which is one of optimal health and life.

While other professions are concerned with changing the environment to suit the weakened body, chiropractic is concerned with strengthening the body to suit the environment.
— B.J. Palmer, DC

CHIROPRACTIC ART

Look well into the spine, for many diseases have their origin in dislocations of the vertebral column.
— Hippocrates

Chiropractic is an art. A chiropractic treatment begins with a diagnosis, the patient's complete history, and determining the onset of symptoms. Chiropractors use their hands to feel the motion of the vertebrae in its range of motion, and then to correct the abnormal structure by giving an adjustment with their hands to that area with the different techniques they were taught in chiropractic school. Just like an artist uses a paintbrush, pencils, or crayons to express his or her talent, the chiropractor uses postural abnormality as a clue to diagnosing the patient's condition. Chiropractors know that abnormal posture plays a major role in a patient's health because it decreases optimal health by causing the body's physiology to change due to the tensions it exerts on particular muscles or joints in the body. Postural abnormality could cause such symptoms as neck pain, temporomandibular (TMJ) headaches, and muscle spasms.

So how do you get abnormal posture? Birth trauma is the most common cause. The birth canal may be too small for the baby or the baby may be breached, or when the doctor is in a rush, the baby is quickly pulled out of the canal, leaving bruises on the baby's shoulders or head. How about such instruments as forceps or the use of suction to help the baby out? These devices cause trauma to the baby and can leave indentations in the skull which later cause such symptoms as migraine headaches. Other possible causes for abnormal postures are slipping and falling, school backpacks (usually when carried on one shoulder), and car accidents. A lot of things we do in our day-to-day activities can cause our body to be out of alignment.

Chiropractors are trained to look for abnormalities in the posture such as a head that is forward, one shoulder being higher than the other, the head tilted to one side, the face being rotated, or a hip that is twisted or is higher on one side than the other. These abnormalities are clues the body leaves for the chiropractor's skilled eyes and hands to detect, and they indicate that a particular area of the body is either over-stimulated or under-stimulated in response to the demands of life's daily stress.

Try looking at your posture for yourself. Look at yourself in the mirror or look at your family members. Compare your image to the image below. Which category do you fall under?

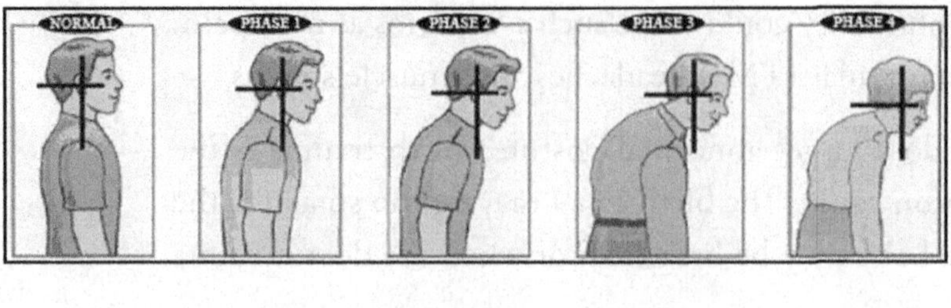

To understand fully the value of chiropractic artwork, we must understand how the body is wired. The body's two most important vital organs are the brain and spinal cords. The brain is the body's main switchboard, and the spinal cord is the highway for all communication. Every move and function in the body is the result of this communication highway. When you pick up a glass of water to drink, it requires your brain to send signals to your hand and fingers to activate the muscles and joints to pick up the glass of water to drink. We pick up the glass naturally without thinking about the process because our body is so amazing. Similar communications happen every second to our vital organs, including the liver, heart, lungs, intestines, and bladder, and each of these vital organs has a major role to play to keep us alive and functioning daily.

Let's look at the body's largest organ, the liver, as an example. The liver is located on the body's right side directly below the diaphragm and protected by the ribs. Some of the liver's major functions are to break down fat, convert glucose into glycogen, and produce urea. But its most important function is to filter out toxic substances in the blood, such as alcohol. The liver also is a place for vitamin and mineral storage, it maintains normal blood glucose levels, and it is responsible for producing 80 percent of the body's cholesterol.

The next most important organ is the heart. We all know that our lives depend upon the heart working. The reason is that our heart is responsible for pumping blood into our lungs to get fresh oxygen and nutrients, and for pumping blood out of the heart to the rest of the body to nourish it. The heart is especially important for pumping blood that goes to the brain because the brain demands a great percentage of the blood's oxygen. Without enough oxygen, the brain will signal the heart to pump harder, and if the heart still cannot provide the brain enough nutrients and oxygen, it will continue to request more and more. This cycle can lead to cardiomegaly, meaning enlarged heart muscles, which are not desirable because they require more energy to pump the blood and do not function as well.

The digestive tract's organs are an amazing system; without them we would not be able to eat. The digestive tract runs from our mouth to our esophagus, and then down to the stomach, small intestine, large intestine, rectum, and anus. Aiding the digestive tract is the liver and pancreas, which release digestive juices to aid in breaking down the foods we eat. A healthy digestive tract allows the body to absorb all the vital nutrients we eat so we can maintain our health.

Finally, the most important of all the body's functions is the nervous system. It consists of the peripheral nervous system (PNS) and the central nervous system (CNS). These two systems are the key to our overall health.

The CNS is comprised of the brain and the spinal cord. Imagine an air traffic control scenario with the central control telling each plane when and where to land. Without that connection, the pilot cannot land. The air traffic controller also tells the pilot at what elevation to fly to avoid crashing the plane. In our body, the brain is the control system and the spinal cord is the highway that carries that message. So if a glitch or abnormality occurs in the system, the body experiences disharmony. Take for example actor Christopher Reeve, who broke his first cervical bone when he fell off a horse, leaving him paralyzed.

That first cervical bone is at the beginning of the pathway. So imagine someone driving on the freeway from I-5 North down to Seattle only to find a major accident has happened and the entire freeway is closed down. What happens to the cars that need to get somewhere to take care of things? They don't get to where they need to go. The same situation applies to our bodies. The messages are being produced, but when the body has disharmony, the messengers cannot reach the right part of the body so the information may be lost or altered. Because the body knows how vital the central nervous system is, it builds a concrete wall around it called the skull and spinal vertebrae.

Similarly, the same situation can happen to the PNS. It is connected to the CNS and is composed of two parts: the somatic and autonomic systems. These two functions are responsible for our outward perception of the world. Input collected from our five senses (sight, smell, taste, touch, and hearing) is part of this system.

Imagine this system operating under an environment of constant noise, pollution, and chaos. This environment is what the body must cope with when it is injured, traumatized, medicated, or has structural abnormality. Our body has to compensate somewhere along its path of communication to keep us alive and operating, which means it will stimulate one part of the organs, muscles, or other body parts more than the other. Here is where chiropractors, through their trained hands, palpate the body to discover blockage and to assist the body in removing it. Chiropractors also educate patients about the contributing factors that cause the body's blockage so patients can prevent the situation from recurring.

A cause must be adjusted, corrected, fixed. To cure, you must treat effects, apply something to the results. Therein lies the greatest transforming value of chiropractic; it adjusts causes, but does not treat effects.

— B.J. Palmer, DC

Chiropractors do not heal the patient's body; they only assist the body in removing the interferences, and once those interferences are removed, the body's natural response is to return to balance. That is why we chiropractors believe, "The power that made the body, heals the body." We believe that our body possesses a very unique quality that allows us to respond to all kinds of stimuli. If given the right environment, the body will return to homeostasis. It likes nothing more than to be in balance.

Therefore, chiropractors analyze and diagnose a patient based on sound medical findings, and then they use their training and skills to correct abnormalities found along the spine in order to help the body return to normal homeostasis.

CHIROPRACTIC SCIENCE

Only 15% of all medical procedures are scientifically validated.

— David Eddy, MD., Ph.D.

Science: Latin word meaning "knowledge." A body of knowledge must stand up to repeated testing by independent observers. — Wikipedia.com

Knowledge: as in facts or principles, knowledge gained by systematic study — Webster's Dictionary

Chiropractic science is based solely on human anatomy

and the body's functions. Chiropractors are trained to detect and diagnose abnormal structures through palpations, leg length analysis, postural abnormality, etc. to determine the actual causes of the patients' pain and symptoms. Once the subluxation(s) have been detected and corrected, the nervous system is free to communicate and flow without any interruption. Chiropractors understand the cause of nerve interference on overall health, and that by removing the interferences, normal function of the nerve will return. Thus, chiropractic science is founded on the fact that vertebral misalignment along the spinal columns and in the cranium is the cause of the patient's pain and symptoms. Chiropractic science understands and addresses the questions of "Why, How, and Where?" Chiropractic adjustment is specific, and its results can be repeated over and over by different chiropractors with the same outcome. This reason is why you hear miracle stories in every chiropractic office around the world.

"Chiropractic is the only science that exactly locates the cause of the dis-ease, then adjusts it."

— BJ Palmer, DC

Chapter 12

CHIROPRACTIC EDUCATION

Chiropractors are required to go through the same prerequisites as medical doctors before they are accepted into chiropractic school. Once in school, chiropractic students take the same courses as medical students, except chiropractic students spend more hours studying in anatomy, physiology, neurology, x-ray, and orthopedics. While in some areas such as psychology, obstetrics, and gynecology, medical students take more hours, ultimately, chiropractic students have more hours of education than medical students. The chart below illustrates the hours of study by chiropractic students vs. medical students.

Table 1. Comparisons of the Overall Curriculum Structure for Chiropractic and Medical Schools

	Chiropractic Schools		Medical Schools	
	Mean	%	Mean	%
Total Contact Hours	4822	100%	4667	100%
Basic science hours	1416	29%	1200	26%

Clinical science hours	3406	71%	3467	74%
Chiropractic science hours	1975	41%	0	0
Clerkship hours	1405	29%	3467	74%

Source: Center for Studies in Health Policy, Inc., Washington, DC. Personal communication of 1995 unpublished data from Meredith Gonyea, PhD

Table 2: Comparison of Hours of Basic Sciences Education in Medical and Chiropractic Schools

Subject	Chiropractic Schools		Medical Schools	
	Hours	% Total	Hours	% Total
Anatomy	570	40	368	31
Biochemistry	150	11	120	10
Microbiology	120	8	120	10
Public Health	70	5	289	24
Physiology	305	21	142	12
Pathology	205	14	162	14
Total Hours	**1,420**	**100**	**1,200**	**100**

Source: Center for Studies in Health Policy, Inc., Washington, DC. Personal communication of 1995 unpublished data from Meredith Gonyea, PhD.

After completion of the required hours and classes, chiropractic students are ready to go into a clinic setting. Chiropractic students get their internships in an outpatient clinic and put in at least 900 hours, while medical students do their internships in hospital settings. Following the completion of chiropractic school, chiropractic students must pass four sections of written and oral National Board Exams before they can then take the state exams and be allowed to practice.

TYPES OF CHIROPRACTIC SERVICE

What differentiated Picasso from Michelangelo or Monet as an artist? His individual technique. Just as a painter may use many different brushes and colors to create his signature artwork, different chiropractors will use different techniques to help their patients. And just as some artists paint with oils while others use watercolors, chiropractors have many different approaches to treatment of the patient's spine.

Each chiropractor is unique in his or her own practice, but all have the common goal for the patient to receive the benefits of the adjustment and to experience the miracle of the body at work. Walk into any chiropractor's office and you will hear story after story of patients who were treated for an ailment and experienced a miracle happening to them. Their first-hand experiences then make these patients walking advertisements for their chiropractors. For that precise reason, chiropractic has been able to stand the test of time for over a century and continues to grow stronger than ever.

Traditional forms of treatment basically consist of hands-on techniques where you tend to hear a bone pop. Some of these traditional techniques are the Gonstead Technique, Diversified Technique, Thompson, Upper Cervical (Toggle), and Leander, which are all hands-on types of treatment.

Newer techniques allow chiropractors to use either their hands or instruments that also work great on the body. Newer versions of chiropractic adjustment are NUCA, BEST, SOT, Activator, CSI, and Brimhall. These are all light force, high velocity techniques.

All of these techniques are effective, so it is the chiropractor's personal choice which one he or she feels most comfortable practicing. Dr. Brimhall's protocol is the most up-to-date technique in terms of combining nutrition, acupuncture, electromagnetic field disturbances, and detoxification of the body with chiropractic. Other practitioners, such as Dr. Ken Best, incorporate Applied Kinesiology (AK) with chiropractic. Practitioners who use the CSI technique are very successful at getting instant results, particularly in helping the patient experience an immediate improvement in his or her ability to breathe. Patients who undergo CSI treatment also find that their flexibility improves greatly.

All in all, any kind of chiropractic adjustment will work. It is all a matter of what level of service you want from your chiropractor and how involved you allow your chiropractor to be in your health.

After all, chiropractors wear many hats in assisting their patients with their health and wellness. They are your health and wellness coaches by educating you about the proper way to exercise and why you need to exercise. They are nutritionists who help you to understand the basic foundation of living a healthy life through eating healthy foods, and they are doctors who will diagnose and treat your ailments by assisting your body to remove its blockages.

Chapter 13

HOW EFFECTIVE IS CHIROPRACTIC TREATMENT?

The doctor of the future will give no medicine,
but will instruct his patient in the care of the human frame, in diet,
and in the cause and prevention of disease.
– Thomas A. Edison

When over 100,000 Americans die each year from medical error, and that number continues to rise, it is understandable that people are looking for alternative ways to treat their ailments. As patients become more informed and educated about their conditions and their overall health, they want to work with providers who are able to deliver the desired results and who are accountable for those treatments.

Chiropractic has the strongest outcome in accountability and results. According to a University of Washington study, as many as 50 percent of all back surgeries are unnecessary or ineffective. A three-year study in Great Britain compared traditional approaches to remedying back pain with chiropractic treatment. The study concluded, "…even after several years, chiropractic was more effective than care provided by medical clinics."

A study done by the State of Florida in 1998 showed a 50 percent reduction in workers' compensation costs and lost work time when chiropractic care was used instead of traditional medical treatment. Another study done by Oregon Worker's Compensation revealed that those who underwent chiropractic care recovered twice as fast as those who sought out traditional medical approaches.

The Agency for Health Care Policy and Research (AHCPR), after countless controlled randomized clinical trials, concluded that treatments for restoration of spinal biomechanics, using methods like those used by chiropractic doctors, were both helpful and highly recommended.

And in the Manga Report, a Canadian research study concluded that approaches employed by chiropractic doctors were more effective than traditional forms of treatment. In fact, they found that the most commonly used medical treatments were often of questionable value.

Finally, Hertzman-Miller et al., in a 2002 issue of the *American Journal of Public Health*, published a study revealing that patients with back pain were more satisfied with chiropractic care than they were with medical care after four weeks of treatment, and more satisfied with chiropractic care than physical therapy after six weeks of treatment.

IS CHIROPRACTIC SAFE?

To appreciate how safe chiropractic treatment is for you and your family, lets look at some statistics regarding the number of deaths attributed to conventional medicine every year. According to the *Journal of the American Medical Association*, "Drug reactions kill 100,000 every year with 2.1 million seriously injured."

Also, in an article in *Life Extension Magazine* titled "Death by Medicine," a group of researchers found that medicine frequently causes more harm than good. And Dr. Richard Besser of the CDC said, "7.5 million unnecessary medical and surgical procedures are performed annually in the US, while approximately 8.9 million Americans are hospitalized unnecessarily."

Furthermore, a recent study by HealthGrades (April 8, 2008) reported that 238,337 potentially preventable error-induced deaths occurred from 2004-2006 in the United States.

Furthermore, as more Americans lose their health insurance from job loss or simply not being able to afford it, they try to treat their pain with over-the-counter (OTC) medication. Every year, people take aspirin, ibuprofen, muscle relaxers, and other pain relief drugs, but these medications only cover up symptoms while ignoring their underlying causes, which can have severe consequences, including death. According to the *Journal of the American Medical Association*, more than 100,000 people die each year from toxic reactions to prescription and OTC drugs. And patients who use OTCs as pain medications are more prone to develop chronic pain syndrome. By comparison, chiropractic care is much safer than taking drugs.

Americans are more aware today that they are better off staying away from a hospital whenever they can because the statistics of unnecessary deaths are so alarming. Even Boeing Vice President of Human Affairs Doug Kight admitted, "You are twenty thousand times more likely to be injured in a hospital than to be injured on a commercial airplane." While commercial airplane mishaps get a lot of publicity, estimates suggest that fewer than 300 people will die this year from flying on commercial aircraft. That means, airplanes are relatively safe, yet chiropractic is much safer than flying.

Still not convinced? According to *The Manga Report*, "One of the most persuasive findings was the issue of safety. The study concluded that chiropractic care is safer than medical management of low back pain." And a New Zealand government investigation into chiropractic care found chiropractic to be "remarkably safe."

Finally, the AHCPR panel, consisting of medical doctors, osteopaths, nurses, physical therapists, and others familiar with the treatment of low back pain, concluded, "relief of pain can be accomplished most safely with nonprescription medication and/or spinal manipulation."

These statistics are evidence that chiropractic is very safe, and no one should be scared of chiropractic treatment. In fact, chiropractic care should be part of your family's healthcare as a preventative approach; visiting a chiropractor will also help to reduce the country's rising costs of healthcare. If people would get regular spinal checkups just like they regularly get their teeth cleaned, we could all save a lot of money on healthcare expenditure and many unfortunate deaths could be prevented.

Go to any chiropractor's office and ask to speak to the patients if you're still not convinced. You'll probably be provided with a list of patients' personal testimonials. Here are just a few from my office:

"I had the good fortune of being referred to Dr. Jeudi Boulom for chiropractic treatments by my friend after a car accident. I was experiencing pain in my shoulder and back to the point that I could not sit or stand for more than ten minutes. After the chiropractic treatment, I experienced tremendous improvement. I felt healthier and experienced a free flow of energy. It was as if the blockage between my mind and body had vanished. I feel so much better—my attitude is definitely better because the pain is gone. There are not enough words to express my thanks and gratitude for the healing hands of my chiropractor." **— Yvonne O.**

"A very severe car accident left me in moderate to extreme pain for several years. My injuries not only included a closed head injury and lacerated spleen, but I also had a compression fracture in my spine and eight broken ribs. Since the accident, the burning nerve pain has been horrible, and I have also suffered with muscle spasms and pain in my mid and lower back and neck. Beginning with my first visit to Dr. Jeudi, I noticed a difference between her and the physical therapists and the acupuncturist I had seen previously. Dr. Jeudi *really* cares, and I could tell she had a strong desire to help me not only to feel better, but also to heal. Just imagine my surprise and delight when after only one session, I felt pain relief I hadn't felt for years. I had been so "locked-up" for so long that I didn't believe anything could help. I believe my positive results with Dr. Jeudi will have a profound impact on my life, and I look forward to being able to do some of the things I have not been able to do for many years." — ***Beth Piasecki***

"My friends and I were in Vancouver, Canada for vacation when a car hit our Honda van. Right after the accident, I suffered severe headaches and neck and lower back pain. I ignored my pain and continued my daily routine until I was not able to bend my back. My head felt heavy and dizzy everyday. My friend introduced me to Dr. Jeudi Boulom. After the first treatment, my head felt much lighter and the dizziness was gone. After a few treatments, I was back to normal and pain free. I would highly recommend Dr. Jeudi to all of my friends." — **Kim O.**

"My experience with chiropractic had been life changing. If it weren't for Dr. Jeudi Boulom educating me on the importance of chiropractic and holistic healthcare, my overall health could have been much worse. Before I had chiropractic care, I had a bad case of gastritis and also ulcers in my stomach that caused excruciating pain almost everyday. Medications that were used to treat my condition were costly and only provided temporary relief, and my family doctor said the medications were the only thing that could help me. But they never solved my problems! I sought out a second opinion and Dr. Jeudi was my last stop. Somehow, for some unbelievable reason, chiropractic adjustments have helped to cure my gastritis and ulcers! Yes! I know, it's hard to see the correlation between spinal adjustments and ulcers, but that's what happened. On top of chiropractic adjustments, Dr. Jeudi informed me about nutritional supplements and ways I could benefit from them. I threw away all of my medications even though my mom thought I was crazy, and I think even my family doctor was surprised when I told him my medical condition was gone. Dr. Jeudi genuinely took my health into consideration and patiently educated me on my health. What I learned has stayed with me ever since. I am grateful to have found her." — **Lili Dang**

Another great testimonial I received was from a young woman in her early thirties who came into the clinic crying and feeling hopeless. She was frantically looking for solutions for her pain and having dreams of seeing deceased ancestors. She went to the ER several times, but no one there could find the source of her complaints. They gave her some medication, but her situation only got worse. So she finally came to our clinic. Here is what she says about the results:

> "I was in such pain that I was hallucinating. I went to the ER several times, but there was nothing they could do except prescribe me pain medication. I thought I was dying until I went to see Dr. Jeudi. She was able to see me even after hours. Immediately after my first treatment, I thought that I had been saved by an angel. Dr. Jeudi truly is my angel. Now, I tell everyone at work to go see Dr. Jeudi and give chiropractic a try. Thanks, Dr. Jeudi." — **V.H.**

Another of my patients had known about chiropractic for years. When he first came to me, he was in his forties and suffering from terrible allergies. He would go through a Costco boxes of Kleenex every month, and his nose was always red and his eyes itchy. He came to see me without his wife knowing because she worked at a hospital where she had heard horror stories about chiropractic, so she had warned her husband never to visit a chiropractor. His allergies were so severe that he decided to give chiropractic care a chance anyway. After just two treatments, his allergies were gone. Later, he convinced his wife to come see me because she was suffering from severe constipation; she had actually passed out twice and had to be taken to the ER while straining to pass a stool. Again, after just a couple of treatments, she experienced relief from her conditions and became a walking advertisement for me.

Finally, as one last example, I had a woman in her early twenties come to see me who was suffering from severe migraine headaches. After a few treatments with chiropractic adjustment, she was freed from her migraines. I moved away soon after that, but years later, we met at a seminar in Fremont, Washington where she told me she had been looking for me all that time just to thank me for relieving her of her migraines.

So what makes chiropractic care so safe and so effective? Chiropractic doesn't add anything into the body like drugs do, and it does not remove anything out of the body like surgery. It honors your body's wisdom and your inborn potential to be healthy. The results patients experience are due to the flow of energy. Our body knows that without restriction or blockage, it will function at its maximum potential. The chiropractor removes blockage from the body so its information highway is free to work as it was designed, thus providing optimal health.

Life constantly bombards us with all kinds of stress, whether it's a family member's death or crises we see in the world such as the recent earthquake in Haiti or the economic meltdown. Losing a job, being unable to feed the family, constant exposure to toxins, a lack of exercise, and unhealthy eating habits all create stress that puts a burden on our organs and our body as a whole. We put such high demands on our body, and yet we spend very little time or money investing in this amazing machine. Instead, we spend money on something that can be easily replaced if it breaks down—but we cannot replace our bodies. Therefore, having regular spinal checkups done by a chiropractor will allow the chiropractor to diagnose and treat the blockages and restore the body to balance without the compromise of medical side effects. This difference is what has helped millions of chiropractic patients and produced high levels of patient satisfaction and safety.

Chiropractic is the largest, most regulated, and best recognized of all the complementary and alternative medicine (CAM) professions. CAM patient surveys show that chiropractors are visited more often than any other alternative provider group and patient satisfaction with chiropractic care is very high. According to an article by Meeker and Haldeman in a 2002 issue of the *Annals of Internal Medicine*, "There is a steadily increasing patient use of chiropractic in the United States, which has tripled in the past two decades."

COST EFFECTIVENESS

In a country where 16 percent of the GDP is spent on healthcare alone, it is obvious that we need to look closely at how we can bring down the cost of healthcare. Especially during this time of economic hardship, everyone is tightening his or her financial belts. Companies are looking at ways to help their employees stay healthy to reduce the red ink in their overall company expenses. For example, Boeing Vice President Doug Kight stated, "Total company revenues last year were $61.5 billion. And in 2006, we spent $1.9 billion of that on health care. Three out of every $100 of revenue is spent on health care for our employees, families, and retirees. So this is a very, very, significant line item."

According to Life Extension Online (www.Lef.org), money spent on healthcare in the U.S. was, "$1.6 trillion in 2003, representing 14% of GDP, considering this enormous expenditure; we should have the best medicine in the world. We should be preventing, and reversing disease, and doing minimal harm. Careful and objective review, however, shows we are the opposite." And Watson Wyatt Worldwide reported, "the average U.S. company spends 6.1 percent of its total annual payroll on sick pay, workers, compensation and disability costs."

How does chiropractic compare to traditional medicine in terms of cost effectiveness? The British National Health Service's research concluded that, "reduced absenteeism could save millions in lost production each year." Because of its effectiveness and long-term benefits, the study recommended that including chiropractic in the British National Health Service should be considered.

Based on *The Manga Report*, Canadian researchers concluded, "Chiropractic care would save hundreds of millions of dollars annually with regard to work disability payments and direct health care costs."

In 1992, the Virginia Research Study concluded, "if chiropractic care was insured to the extent of other medical specialties, it would likely emerge as a first option for many patients with certain medical conditions. They also believed this could result in a decrease in overall treatment costs for these conditions."

HOW EFFECTIVE IS CHIROPRACTIC TREATMENT?

In June 1993, with a follow-up in September 1994, the *Journal of Manipulative and Physiological Therapeutics* reported on "a retrospective study of statistical analysis comparing insurance costs (payouts) for people with one or more of 493 neuro-musculoskeletal diagnostic codes, done by Professor Miron Stano at Oakland University in Rochester, Michigan." The study included nearly 400,000 patients and both the original study and the follow-up showed "people receiving chiropractic care experienced 30% lower health care costs than those receiving medical care only."

Given that American health insurance continues to rise and that over 50 million Americans are without insurance, the savings involved, as demonstrated by all this research, and the improved health and welfare of people as the result of chiropractic care would be a tremendous benefit to the U.S. government, U.S. businesses, and the American people as a whole.

Chapter 14

WHY A CHIROPRACTOR?

Why search the world over for an exterminator or an antidote for dis-ease? Why not look for the cause of the ailments in the person affected and then correct it?

— BJ Palmer, DC

Our body is an amazing machine that can perform many magical things we want it to do. For instance, if you cut yourself, your body responds instantly with the healing mechanism by first stopping the bleeding and then sealing the area from further bleeding, and it guards the body from any possible infection. Our body does all this without our command. It just knows what to do. However, our body requires that we supply it with the proper nutrients, and it also requires that the communication highway is free of restriction so it can carry out its job.

Let's go back to our car analogy for a minute. When the red light comes on saying our car needs service, do you put tape over the light so you can ignore it? Taking medication for our pain is like putting tape over our car's warning light. It does not tell us the reason for the pain. When that warning light comes on, you could also just unplug the wire that lights it. That's what we do when we have surgery to remove the problem rather than healing it.

We all know the best thing to do when that warning light comes on is to take the car to the mechanic, so when you have pain symptoms, why wouldn't you go to a chiropractor?

Chiropractic care is safe, effective, and much less expensive than traditional medicine. Today, tens of millions of Americans are losing their health insurance so they are looking for alternative ways to treat chronic conditions. Furthermore, it is pretty clear a change in our healthcare system is needed. As Life Extension Online has said, "It is evident that the American medical system is itself the leading cause of death and injury in the US." The evidence is clear—just look at these statistics:

Estimated Annual Mortality and Economic Cost of Medical Intervention

Condition	**Deaths**	**Cost**
Adverse Drug Reactions	106,000	$ 12 billion
Medical Error	98,000	$ 2 billion
Bedsores	115,000	$55 billion
Infection	88,000	$ 5 billion
Malnutrition	108,000	———
Outpatients	199,000	$ 77 billion
Unnecessary Procedures	37,136	$122 billion

Surgery-Related	32,000	$ 9 billion
Totals:	783,936	$282 billion

Source: *Life Extension Magazine*, www.lef.org

Obviously, these statistics are alarming and prove that alternative forms of healthcare treatment are needed. Therefore, chiropractic treatment is the fourth investment in creating health and wellness for you and your family.

CHIROPRACTIC BENEFITS ALL AGES

As the data I've presented shows, chiropractic treatment can be extremely beneficial. In fact, it is effective for patients of all ages, from infants to senior citizens.

How can chiropractic treatment benefit children? Children are very active so they fall and injure themselves a lot. Children should also be evaluated for abnormal posture as a result of falls, or slouching, or sitting in front of the computer. If left untreated, children might develop joint diseases like arthritis or experience such symptoms as headaches and tiredness, or frequent illnesses like ear infections, allergies, and retarded physical development because of nerve impingement which over long periods of time can lead to abnormal functions in the body, just as a bent twig will grow into a crooked tree.

Furthermore, children need chiropractic care because birth trauma is the number one cause of spinal misalignment. As stated earlier, forceps or vacuum devices to help pull a baby from the womb can be traumatic to the skull. Statistics show that 1 in every 1,000 babies experiences birth trauma, resulting in cranial nerve injuries, brachial plexus injuries, cerebral palsy, head injuries, or other peripheral nerve injuries. Birth trauma ranges each year from being the sixth to the tenth leading cause of infant mortality in the United States.

Senior citizens are great candidates for chiropractic treatment because as we age, we tend to lose our ability to move. And since life is a result of motion, our health can be diminished by a lack of it. Chiropractic helps senior citizens move again with chiropractic treatments and adjunctive therapy. The treatments increase the nerve function, which allows the body to perform the daily activities of living with minimal or no pain. A Swedish study proves that chiropractic care over a period of two or more years helps the cells to repair DNA, which actually makes you healthier.

Chiropractic is great for patients with work, sports, or automobile accident injuries because chiropractors support the proper healing of the body. The body starts the healing process within the first seventy-two hours of injury, but if not healed properly, the body will heal with scar tissues. Scar tissues are one of the greatest limitations to achieving optimal health because they cause continual pain and sap energy from your body.

Even active individuals who are currently healthy and have no symptoms should have their spines evaluated by a chiropractor to make sure there is no restricted flow of life. As I've said before, we take a car to the mechanic every so many miles for an oil change or tire rotation to make our car last longer. We don't wait for our car to break down to take care of it, so we should give that same level of preventive care to our bodies. For healthy individuals, getting your spine "tune-up" on a regular basis is an essential and wise investment.

Celebrities are often obsessed with taking care of their health, and chiropractors have long been popular among them. Actors like Bob Hope, Alan Thicke, Demi Moore, and Bruce Willis have all had their own personal chiropractors. Musicians who visit chiropractors include Mindi Abiar, Jessey J, the members of Chicago, and Bon Jovi; they especially see their chiropractors before they put on a concert.

I probably don't even have to tell you how popular chiropractic is among professional athletes, including Joe Montana, Regi Miller, Troy Aikman, Emmitt Smith, Jerry Rice, and many more. These athletes understand the value and the role chiropractic plays in their overall health and performance. Another great example is Lance Armstrong; he has his own chiropractor with him every time he races the Tour de France.

Chiropractic benefits patients from all walks of life, from special needs patients to healthy patients. Everyone should get his or her spine evaluated by a chiropractor, not only for aches and pain, but to maintain a healthy body. Remember, pain is the first clue the body gives to let us know that something is wrong, and no one can diagnose the problem better than an expert mechanic of the body—your chiropractor. Thus, the fourth investment for creating a healthy life is getting regular chiropractic checkups.

Section 5

HOW CHANGE AND LEADERSHIP AFFECT YOUR HEALTH

*We must learn to view change as a natural phenomenon—
to anticipate it and to plan for it. The future is ours to channel in the
direction we want to go...we must continually ask ourselves,
"What will happen if...?" or better still, "How can we make it happen?"*
– Lisa Taylor

Chapter 15

CHANGE YOUR LIFESTYLE

Imagine life as a game in which you are juggling five balls in the air. You name them—work, family, health, friends, and spirit—and you're keeping all of these in the air. You will soon understand that work is a rubber ball. If you drop it, it will bounce back. But the other four balls—family, health, friends, and spirit are made of glass. If you drop one of these, they will be irrevocably scuffed, marked, nicked, damaged, or even shattered. They will never be the same. You must understand that and strive for balance in your life.

– Brian Dyson, CEO of Coca Cola Enterprises from 1959-1994

Life is a result of constant changes, and change is good for all life forms. For example, the weather changes every week from being sunny to raining or snowing, and from hot to cold. The caterpillars change their forms into beautiful butterflies. The days change into nights, and the clouds change the sky from blue to gray. If we look around us, we see constant changes happening everyday. Nothing stays the same.

For many of us, change occurs when a need or desire exists for something different from what we are used to everyday or from what is affecting our lives negatively. Let me give you a few examples of some changes that have happened, many of which were difficult, but which have resulted in many benefits in the long run. They all can be seen as analogies of the positive change we can make by investing in our health.

Most Americans thought that after eight years under President George W. Bush, with the economy going bankrupt, people without jobs, and homes being lost, they were ready for a change, so they elected Barack Obama as president because his campaign slogan "CHANGE WE NEED" promised what they wanted. Although everyone may not agree with the changes President Obama has made, he has definitely been fulfilling his promise to bring about change.

Think of the Wright brothers—they changed the way we travel. People used to say about the Wright brothers, "They seem like well-meaning, decent young men. Yet there they are, neglecting their business to waste their time, day after day, on that ridiculous flying machine." But the Wright brothers defied all pessimistic people and proved that if you keep working and practicing, you will accomplish your goals. Nothing is ridiculous or impossible if we are willing to make the changes in our life necessary to make it happen.

My dad made a change in our lives after we survived the holocaust in Cambodia. He saw the life that we were living, and he saw a better future for us, so he saved up some money and then hired a special tour guide to take us out of Cambodia and into the border of Thailand. It was a very scary time in our lives. We had to hide and run in the night to avoid being caught by both the Khmer Rouge soldiers and the Thai soldiers at the border. But despite the risk involved, including the possibility of our being killed, my dad wanted a better future for us all so he made the decision to leave our homeland. My dad changed our lives by taking us out of a country recently devastated by its worst war and bringing us to the United States, a country full of opportunity and abundance. After my older sister and I reunited with our dad following the war in Cambodia, he hired a man who knew his way to the Thailand border, to lead us to Thailand. And from there my dad somehow contacted our relatives in the United States who had been fortunate enough to leave the country before the fall of the Cambodia. Our sponsors, Connie and Woody Uy, lived in Yakima, Washington, so we first lived there in the United States.

Just as my father wanted a better future for his children, Dr. Martin Luther King Jr. wanted a better world for his children and all African Americans. In leading marches to Washington D.C. to ask for an end to segregation laws, he helped to change a nation, making it move from prejudice to greater freedom and equality for everyone. Not only did he risk his life to bring about this change for the better, but he made the ultimate sacrifice when he was assassinated, becoming a martyr for his beliefs and efforts.

In my own life, I've personally had to make changes to improve a situation. When I was in high school, I worked part-time at a grocery store in Seattle as a cashier for my dad's friend. I enjoyed working there because the boss and I had a great relationship, and we would joke and laugh together as if we were family. I was trusted enough that they gave me the key to the cash box so I could make change for large bills when customers paid. However, one busy day, my two bosses and I all made change from the cash box. At the end of the day, the bosses counted the money and realized they were short $1,000. That's a lot of money, and it was even more so back in the 1980s. After they told me they were short the money, they asked me whether I knew what could have happened. Of course, I felt terrible that they had lost so much money, but I was more concerned when I began to fear they would no longer trust me. During the next few weeks, my fears came true when my bosses started to act very weird. They would sneak around and spy on what I was doing, and they even installed a surveillance camera that pointed at the cash register. It was a very awkward time, so I decided to quit working where I wasn't trusted, and instead, I found work at the 7-Eleven closer to my house.

Another example of change occurred when we first moved to Seattle and my dad was still looking for a job. He rented an apartment at Graham Street and Rainier Avenue, which was all he could afford at the time. We had no idea what we were getting ourselves into there. While living in that apartment, we witnessed all sorts of crime. The first time was when my little brother and two older cousins went to play basketball at the park nearby; they were jumped and beaten up by a high school football team. Their assailants also smashed up my cousin's car after he refused to give them the gold necklace he was wearing. All three came home with bruises and bloody mouths. The second time was when my younger siblings were playing outside the door of the apartment building. I had just sat down to watch the "The Care Bears" when one of my sisters came to tell me that a man had snatched our sister's necklace. When we went and tried to ask her how it had happened, all we got was constant screaming. Later, I learned that the man had somehow lured her to come near the stairway where he was able to snatch the necklace from her neck. The third incident happened when we were all asleep; a burglar came into our apartment and took my aunt's purse. She had $150 in her purse that she was going to use to buy her two-month old daughter's baby formula. After we called the police, we learned that the entire apartment complex had been burglarized. Finally, the incident that really made my dad want to move was when my younger brother's grades were slipping and he was getting into trouble with the law. Furthermore, my brother was scared to take the garbage out because our neighbor who lived on the floor below us had stabbed his wife nine times and killed her. After that incident, my brother was scared to walk down the stairs alone; instead, he would toss the garbage down from the third floor. All these incidents led to my father deciding we had to change our living environment for a better one. We moved up north to Mountlake Terrace, and soon after, my brother made tremendous changes in his academic and personal behavior, going from being a D- to a straight A student, and getting involved in school sports.

My point with all of these examples is that sometimes our situations are difficult—we may even feel that we are stuck without any hope of a way out, but if we take the time to assess what is important, we can make the changes necessary. If you think about it, I'm sure you can think of past times in your own life when you were afraid to change something, but when you finally took the risk, the resulting benefits were well worth it, and you are now glad you made that change.

Today, we are all well aware that our healthcare system and our personal levels of health are badly in need of change. Statistics from 2006 show that nine out of ten workers live with chronic pain, and that's nearly a 40 percent increase from 1996. Plus, 23.6 million Americans have been diagnosed with diabetes, and 45 million Americans are seriously affected each year by headaches. It is clear that as a whole, the American people are sick and in need of change. And, although the CDC and both the federal and local state governments are looking for ways to make Americans healthier, we as individuals need to participate and take responsibility for making a change in our family's lifestyle.

Why not start by making changes at home? Why not take your health into your own hands and make the lifestyle changes necessary to improve your health, especially if you are tired of living in pain and want to do something about it? I believe if the American people change their ways of eating, sleeping, and living, we will all be much healthier.

I've learned to practice what I preach regarding making my own changes in healthcare. For example, who doesn't want to look young and have beautiful skin? If you've ever had eczema, or acne like I've had, you know how much you wish you had beautiful skin. Since our skin is the by-product of what we put into our bodies, why not change the way we live by eating healthier foods, by exercising to release toxins, by avoiding toxic products, and by getting regular spinal checkups?

I didn't realize the dramatic effects that food can have on our bodies until I entered my late thirties. That was when I started to notice I was getting paler and more wrinkles were starting to appear on my face. When I was younger, I would go out in public without worrying about wearing makeup, but as my body became more and more deficient in nutrients and lower in energy, I needed makeup so I would look half-decent. However, as I started to change my way of eating by consuming more raw and organic vegetables and getting more hours of sleep, I noticed my energy starting to come back. Now my skin has more color and looks younger and more alive. I especially have noticed the change in my lips, which now look pinker without my having to apply lipstick to them. Plus, I can now get up without feeling the aches and the stiffness I used to feel every morning.

You might say, "You're a doctor, so how can you be suffering like that?" But I am as human as everyone else. When I neglect my body yet demand a lot from it, my energy gauge becomes low. By not feeding my body the right kind of nutrients, I created a poor intestinal lining for myself, which basically cut years off of my life. Fortunately, by feeding my body proper nutrients, exercising, avoiding toxic substances, and getting regular spinal care, I can reverse most of the damage.

Being physically fit, having more energy, losing weight—all these situations can be achieved just by making simple changes to how we eat and live. When we take proper care of our bodies, the pain goes away, the acne disappears, and the weight comes off. You end up energized and with beautiful, young, and radiant skin. Therefore, I challenge you to take action today and change your family's way of eating, sleeping, communicating, and exercising. Old habits are always hard to change, but if you persist, healthy new habits will eventually seem natural and the benefits will make the difficulties seem small by comparison.

EXERCISES

What areas of your life need change?

____

How can you make those areas better?

____

What health issues do you have now that can use some change?

____

Chapter 16

TAKE THE LEADERSHIP ROLE IN YOUR LIFE

People find themselves in leadership roles through circumstances. As Malvolio might have put it: some are born leaders, some achieve positions of leadership whilst others have leadership thrust upon them.

— **Sir Liam Donaldson,** speaking on medical leadership at Keele University, 24th January 2002

What is a leader? To me, a leader is someone who has a clear, strong vision of where he or she wants to go. Leaders are those who can passionately and clearly communicate their thoughts and get things done by inspiring others to help bring about their visions.

An example of great leadership is President John F. Kennedy. At age forty-three, he was the youngest president ever elected, and he had many great visions for the future of the United States and its people. In his inaugural speech, he said, "Ask not what your country can do for you; ask what you can do for your country." Among President Kennedy's visions was that the

U.S. would be first to land on the moon—a dream that became reality on July 20, 1969. President Kennedy also envisioned a life of equality for African-Americans so he helped to pass new laws that ended discrimination. Furthermore, President Kennedy led our country out of danger during the Cuban Missile Crisis when he demanded that the Russians remove their weapons from Cuba. He also had a clear goal of peace around the world that led to his creating the Peace Corps, an organization whose volunteers travel to other countries to help them find solutions to their problems and to create a better way of life for their people. According to President Kennedy, the Peace Corps represented, "The kind of peace that makes life on earth worth living…not merely peace for Americans but peace for all men and women." President Kennedy's great leadership is still remembered today, nearly half a century after his death. Because of his great leadership, his burial ground has an eternal flame burning.

Another great leader was President Dwight D. Eisenhower. It was his vision and his leadership that led to the efficient highway system we all use today. President Eisenhower was such a great leader that during his presidency, Americans prospered, and he is credited with creating many jobs for the American people so they could buy single-family homes. The economy was booming during his leadership years. Under his presidency, racial segregation was made unconstitutional and schools were integrated in the South. Also during his presidency, Alaska and Hawaii became states. The American people re-elected President Eisenhower to a second term because of his great leadership and his character. His character had been formed when he was young and he demonstrated it throughout his life first as a successful football coach, then as a military leader who instilled trust and confidence in his staff, and later as a politician who always kept his promises. The American people felt safe during Eisenhower's presidency, and they were optimistic about the livelihood and wellbeing of the nation.

Remember Mother Theresa? Her compassionate love and caring for mankind was so genuine that the leaders of many countries rewarded her for her passion and commitment. She never discriminated against anyone, and she had the greatest compassion for the poor and sick. She gave hope to those who felt hopeless, she instilled love into those who lacked love, and she became the companion to those in need of a friend.

Being a great leader requires that you have the basic foundation of character, vision, and personality. The above examples are of leaders with extraordinary visions for the future of the people they led and who had personalities that people loved, respected, and admired.

Not all leaders are great leaders. Knowing how to recognize a great leader and to follow his or her example can take people far in life, but following the wrong leader can lead to destruction for the people involved.

For example, when I was a little girl in Cambodia, the Khmer Rouge leaders initially had good intentions, but they had poor vision, poor organization, and they lacked the right character traits. The leaders would give orders to the commanders below them, but power-hungry egos and miscommunication resulted in abuse of the people. In the small village where I lived, the village commander was always looking for young children who would spy on their family members and report back to the leaders. They had brainwashed children into believing that anyone who disagreed with the leaders was an enemy to the country and should, therefore, be killed. At night, my family and I would hear the footsteps of people being taken from their homes to be murdered. One night, our neighbor's parents were taken; their daughter screamed her lungs out, and after that, she became incoherent and pretty much crazy as a result of the traumatic experience. It was a very sad and scary time to be alive.

Although, the Khmer Rouge leaders had great intentions for the Cambodian people, their lack of clear vision, personality, and moral character ended up costing the country a lot of pain and millions of innocent lives. Their wish to eliminate the concept of social class so everyone was equal would have worked had they been able to organize the country so food was properly distributed and people were treated properly. Their communication and moral failures ultimately resulted in Cambodia's failure to become a socialist country.

Too often we look to the wrong people to be our leaders. I've been guilty of this myself. In high school, I hung out with a group of my peers who thought it was cool to skip class and instead smoke cigarettes and talk about meaningless stuff. Fortunately, my common sense soon kicked in, and rather than following them, I stayed in class.

Our friends can influence and lead us to do things that are not necessarily good for us or for them. Knowing when to follow and when not to follow is important. We each need to be the leader in our own life, and it takes strength, vision, willpower, and determination to become that person, but it leads us to becoming the person we want to be. We choose to lead ourselves when we take the steps to envision the future and apply our knowledge and determination daily to make that vision come true.

Finally, in the realm of healthy living, I want to remind you of the great example of Jack LaLanne, an athlete and health guru who is still going strong in his nineties. He is known as the "Father of Fitness" because he has led by example. He practices what he teaches every day of his life. He eats fresh fruits and vegetables and he exercises daily. He is an inspiration to us all, and he has paved the way for many more people, including us, to step forward and lead the healthcare revolution by learning how to invest in healthy living.

I believe that now is the time for America to have a strong leader who can take action and get involved in solving our healthcare crisis. We need someone who can stand up against all the challenges and risks and lead the people and the nation toward becoming healthier.

But no leader can accomplish everything alone. Change requires everyone's participation. That means we need to take action and take on the leadership roles in our homes, communities, and states by setting an example for others to follow.

Now is the time to take up the challenge and to lead your family and your country out of the current economic and health crisis by bringing out changes to healthcare, both in the system and in our individual lives. Look deep inside yourself and find the leader inside you. What can you do for your family and your community?

One thing I decided to do to take on a leadership role is to write this book. I hope it will inspire many people to make changes in their and their families' lives so they can be wiser, healthier, and happier.

Another thing I've done is become a chiropractor. In addition, beyond just treating my patients, I spend my time educating them about their bodies so they can take better care of their health. I believe that if we create more awareness about the importance and the value of being healthy, then more people will take care of themselves and less lives will be lost by unnecessary medical errors and over-medication. Ultimately, the nation as a whole will save more money, but most importantly, millions of human lives will be saved and people will experience richer lives in every sense.

No, you don't have to write a book or become a doctor. You can start simply in your own home. Lead your family into a healthy lifestyle by creating a healthy living environment for you and your family. Eat more fruits and vegetables, and plan to exercise as a family by riding bicycles, walking in the park, or going hiking. Remember our children are living examples of who we are. They are inactive because we are; they are overweight because we allow them to be. Parents need to be the leaders in their families. By spending time with your children while exercising, you will make everyone healthier and bring yourself closer together as a family. By sitting down together to eat a healthy meal rather than grabbing fast food, you will cultivate family togetherness centered upon healthy living, and the example is one your children will then pass on to their own children someday. By being leaders in our families, we can bring about change in America.

On a community level, we can bring about change by creating community safety-watch programs so when your family goes out for a walk, it is safe to do so. Have a block party so everyone gets to know each other. Just make sure you bring healthy food to the party to set a good example. Be the first to reach out to your neighbors, and you may then inspire them to reach out to others.

Use your talents to lead your country back to health. If you take on the leadership role and lead by example, others will follow and help you. Soon Americans will be healthy again.

A Final Note

ACHIEVING YOUR OPTIMAL HEALTH

One Flaw In Women

Women have strengths that amaze men…

They bear hardships and they carry burdens,

but they hold happiness, love and joy.

They smile when they want to scream.

They sing when they want to cry.

They cry when they are happy

and laugh when they are nervous.

They fight for what they believe in.

They stand up to injustice.

They don't take "no" for an answer

when they believe there is a better solution.

They go without so their family can have.

They go to the doctor with a frightened friend.

They love unconditionally.

They cry when their children excel

and cheer when their friends get awards.
They are happy when they hear about
a birth or a wedding.
Their hearts break when a friend dies.
They grieve at the loss of a family member,
yet they are strong when they
think there is no strength left.
They know that a hug and a kiss
can heal a broken heart.
Women come in all shapes, sizes and colors.
They'll drive, fly, walk, run or e-mail you
to show how much they care about you.
The heart of a woman is what
makes the world keep turning.
They bring joy, hope and love.
They have compassion and ideas.
They give moral support to their family and friends.
Women have vital things to say and everything to give.
HOWEVER, IF THERE IS ONE FLAW IN WOMEN,
IT IS THAT THEY FORGET THEIR WORTH."
— Anonymous

Achieving your Optimal Health is simply a matter of priorities. Life is full of abundance in all its aspects. Everything is relative. Our health and happiness all depend on how we choose to view and handle our lives.

Health is the key component that determines the quality of

every aspect of our lives and the lives of those we love. Without our health, there is no joy to living. When we are sick, we feel restricted, limited, and sometimes we give up any hope of ever getting back on track and regaining the health we had so we can partake in all the things we love to do.

However, all things are possible when you believe. All possibilities become realities if we are determined to achieve the goals we set for ourselves. Yes, they require time, effort, and commitment, but if we attend to them wisely, anything can be achieved.

Optimal Health can be achieved by applying the four fundamental principles of investing in your health. Here is the formula that will surely give you back your health and the longevity you desire. When this formula is applied daily, the return on your investment is priceless.

NUTRITION
+
EXERCISE
+
DETOXIFICATION
+
<u>CHIROPRACTIC CARE</u>

$ MONEY SAVED $
NO PAIN • LESS STRESS
BETTER SLEEP • MORE ENERGY
WEIGHT LOSS • BEAUTIFUL SKIN
YOUTHFULNESS • LONGEVITY

Your ability to reap the full benefits of this formula depends solely upon how much you are willing to invest in your health. We are all familiar with the financial question "What is your net worth?" Ask yourself what is your net worth in relation to your health? Next, ask yourself what your health is worth? Can a price be set on your health? For my family and me, our health is priceless. I am willing to do everything it takes to make sure that everyone in my family is healthy.

I challenge you to start investing in your health as soon as you finish this book. Life should be free from pain, from limitations or restrictions, and it should be filled with joy, laughter, and the ability to move and go wherever you please. You deserve that joy and pleasure now. Don't wait until the president or Congress or anyone else passes a healthcare bill. Don't wait until you are diagnosed with a terminally ill condition. Don't wait until someone in your family is taken away from you by illness. Don't wait until the healthcare bills become law because that could be three or four years down the road. Start now. Start to create a healthy body for yourself today so you can enjoy your life tomorrow and for many years to come.

Come take this journey with me. Together we will solve the healthcare crisis one person at a time. All obstacles can appear too big to conquer at first, but if we take them one step at a time, eventually they will become easy. Begin your journey of health now, step by step.

Once you start this journey to optimal health, I would love to hear about the amazing things that happen to you and your family. You can contact me at:

www.DrJeudi.com

RECOMMENDED READING

Baillie-Hamilton, Paula. *Stop the 21st Century Killing You.*

Baker, Nena. *The Body Toxic: How the Hazardous Chemistry of Everyday Things Threatens Our Health and Well-Being.*

Batmanghelidj, Fereydoon. *Obesity Cancer Depression: Their Common Cause & Natural Cure.*

Batmanghelidj, **Fereydoon.** *Water Cures, Drugs Kill.*

Batmanghelidj, Fereydoon. *Water for Health, for Healing, for Life: You're Not Sick, You're Thirsty!*

Batmanghelidj, Fereydoon. *Your Body's Many Cries for Water.*

Berg, Eric. *The 7 Principles of Fat Burning: Get Healthy, Lose Weight and Keep It Off!*

Blech, Jorg. *Healing Through Exercise.*

Brantley, Timothy. *The Cure: Heal Your Body, Save Your Life.*

Brimhall, John and Brett Brimhall. *Solving the Health Puzzle with the 6 Steps to Wellness.*

Cherniske, Stephen. *Caffeine Blues: Wake Up to the Hidden Dangers of America's #1 Drug.*

Cherniske, Stephen. *The Metabolic Plan: Stay Younger Longer.*

Emoto, Masaru. *The Healing Power of Water.*

Fife, Bruce. *Coconut Cures: Preventing and Treating Common Health Problems with Coconut.*

Jones, Dennis Merritt. *The Art of Being: 101 Ways to Practice Purpose in Your Life.*

McCarthy, Jenny. *Mother Warriors: A Nation of Parents Healing Autism Against All Odds.*

Miller, Neil Z. *Vaccines: Are They Really Safe and Effective?*

Palmer, D.D. *The Chiropractor.*

Price, Weston F. and Price-Pottenger Nutrition Foundation. *Nutrition and Physical Degeneration.*

Rondberg, Terry A. *Chiropractic First.*

Siegal, Bernie S. *Love, Medicine & Miracles: Lessons Learned About Self-Healing from a Surgeon's Experience with Exceptional Patients.*

Stoll, Walt, Jan DeCourtney and C. Norman Shealy. *Recapture Your Health.*

Sweere, Joseph J. *Golden Rules for Vibrant Health in Body, Mind, and Spirit.*

Trudeau, Kevin. *Natural Cures "They" Don't Want You to Know About.*

Truman, Karol K. *Feelings Buried Alive Never Die…*

Whorton, James C. *Nature Cures: The History of Alternative Medicine in America.*

Wiley, Harvey W. *The History of A Crime Against the Food Law.*

Wilk, Chester A. *Chiropractic Speaks Out.*

ESSENTIAL CHIROWELLNESS CLINIC

The Essential ChiroWellness Clinic was established in June 2009 after many requests from patients who wanted Dr. Jeudi Boulom to return back into practice. After taking a year off to be with her children, she was blessed to see what she wanted to do with her life, and how she could use her talents to help others regain their optimal health.

The mission of Essential ChiroWellness is to be a facility where patients can come in with their conditions and be given the time for an analysis that will result in a treatment plan tailored to fit the individual's true needs. After many years of practice, Dr. Jeudi found that no two individuals are the same and that no two treatments are the same. While many patients come to the clinic believing they just need to have their spines corrected, Dr. Jeudi shows them how to address underlying factors vital to full recovery. Thus, being able to walk her patients through their personal health requirements and what changes will lead to their achievement of overall wellbeing has truly been a blessing for both Dr. Jeudi and her patients. By educating her patients and helping them see what is needed and why they need it, Dr. Jeudi makes it easier for her patients to follow through with her recommendations and to take an active role in improving their health.

Essential ChiroWellness uses the most up-to-date technologies, techniques, and skills. The clinic offers a combination of nutrition education, exercise protocol, detoxification, and spinal health all under one roof.

ABOUT THE AUTHOR

Dr. Jeudi Boulom has been providing quality chiropractic healthcare for over ten years. Her gentle holistic approach and basic natural solutions for many common health issues have improved the lives of numerous Washingtonian citizens. Her chiropractic services are tailored to the needs of each unique patient.

Dr Jeudi's services include a holistic approach based on sound medical knowledge. Her goal is to enhance the quality of life through wellness care with basic solutions.

Dr. Jeudi Boulom received her undergraduate study at Shoreline Community College where she was awarded Woman of the Year. She is a 1996 graduate of Parker College of Chiropractic. Dr. Jeudi is licensed with the Washington State Department of Health to practice chiropractic in the State of Washington. She is a Brimhall Certified Practitioner (having completed the Brimhall 6 Steps to Wellness Protocol training), a Cranial Adjustment Therapy Provider, and a Reiki Certified Practitioner. Dr. Jeudi is multilingual in English, Cambodian, and Laotian.

Dr. Jeudi brings forth unique skills and knowledge that are priceless to her patients. She is passionate about her work and her patients' health and wellbeing. Dr. Jeudi is sincere, and she encourages her patients to be open in order for true healing to flourish.

Dr. Jeudi's activities include mentoring other chiropractors and helping them achieve maximum health and wellness for their patients. Dr. Jeudi has also served as President (2008/2009) of the MLK Business Association, an organization that promotes a prosperous business community along the MLK light-rail corridor.

Most importantly, Dr. Jeudi is the mother of two adorable children who bring her light and joy everyday.

BIBLIOGRAPHY

Chapter 1

1. Baillie-Hamilton, Paula. *Stop the 21st Century from Killing You.* p. 88

2. The Eck Institute of Applied Nutrition and Bioenergetics.

3. Wikipedia.com

4. www.aimforherbs.com/remakingbeets.html

5. www.askdears.com/html/4/t044900.asp

6. www.naturalnews.com/022331_food_American_diet_standard_american_diet.html

7. Metagenics.com

8. Batmanghelidj, **Fereydoon.** *Water Cures, Drugs Kill.*

Chapter 2

1. Cherniske, Stephen. *The Metabolic Plan: Stay Younger Longer.*

2. Wikipedia.com

3. coconutresearchercenter.org

4. Fife, Bruce. *Coconut Cures: Preventing and Treating Common Health Problems with Coconut.*

5. Linus Pauling Institute. http://lpi.oregonstate.edu/infocenter/minerals/calcium/index.html

6. www.buzzle.com/articles/potassium-deficiency-effects-of-low-potassium.html

Chapter 3

1. Wikipedia.com

2. http://health.learninginfo.org/nutrition-facts/cabbage.html

3. www.juicing-for-health.com/cabbage.html

4. http://www.nutritiondata.com/facts/vegetables-and-vegetable-products/2390/2

Chapter 5

1. Blech, Jorg. *Healing Through Exercise.*

2. Cherniske, Stephen. *The Metabolic Plan: Stay Younger Longer.*

3. Cherniske, Stephen. *Caffeine Blues: Wake Up to the Hidden Dangers of America's #1 Drug.*

4. JackLaLanne.com

5. www.obesity.org/statistics

6. Batmanghelidj, **Fereydoon.** *Water Cures, Drugs Kill.*

Chapter 8

1. "The Dark Side of Immunization." *Journal of Science* (Nov 22, 1997).

2. Baker, Nena. *The Body Toxic: How the Hazardous Chemistry of Everyday Things Threatens Our Health and Well-Being.*

3. Baillie-Hamilton, Paula. *Stop the 21st Century Killing You.*

4. Miller, Neil Z. *Vaccines: Are They Really Safe and Effective?*

5. Truman, Karol. *Feelings Buried Alive Never Die…*

Chapter 9

1. Baillie-Hamilton, Paula. *Stop the 21st Century Killing You.*

2. Timothy Brantley, ND. BrantleyCure.com

3. electropollution.org

4. Brimhall, John and Brett Brimhall. *Solving the Health Puzzle with the 6 Steps to Wellness.*

Chapter 10

1. Palmer, D.D. *The Chiropractor.*

2. Whorton, James C. *Nature Cures: The History of Alternative Medicine in America.*

3. Wilk, Chester A. *Chiropractic Speaks Out.*

4. Rondberg, Terry A. *Chiropractic First.*

5. ACAtoday.org

Chapter 11

1. Palmer, D.D. *The Chiropractor.*

2. Rondberg, Terry A. *Chiropractic First.*

3. Sweere, Joseph J. *Golden Rules for Vibrant Health in Body, Mind, and Spirit.*

4. Brimhall, John and Brett Brimhall. *Solving the Health Puzzle with the 6 Steps to Wellness.*

5. Wilk, Chester A. *Chiropractic Speaks Out.*

6. ACAtoday.org

Chapter 12

1. Rondberg, Terry A. *Chiropractic First.*

2. ACAtody.org

3. Nelson, Carl et al. "Manual Healing Diversity and Other Challenges to Chiropractor Integration." Meridianinstitute.com

4. http://chiroweb.com/archives/ahcpr/chapter3.htm

Chapter 13

1. Palmer, D.D. *The Chiropractor.*

2. Lef.org

3. www.who.int/patientsafety/events/media/SSSL_backgnd_paper.pdf

4. "British study endorses chiropractic." *Science* 248 (July 1990): 1610.

5. Eisenberg, DM et al. "Unconventional medicine in the United States: prevalence, costs, and patterns of use." *New England Journal of Medicine* 328 (Jan 28, 1993): 246-52.

6. Jarvis, KB, Phillips, RB, and Morris, EK. "Cost per case comparison of back injury claims of chiropractic versus medical management for conditions with identical diagnostic codes." *Journal of Occupation Medicine* 33.8 (August 1991): 847-52.

7. Koes, BW et al. "Randomized clinical trial of manipulative therapy and physiotherapy for persistent back and neck complaints: results of a one-year follow-up." *British Medical Journal* 304 (March 7, 1992): 601-5.

8. www.silcom.com/~dwsmith/magna.html

9. *British Medical Journal.* (June 2, 1990).

10. "Spinal adjustment for low back pain." www.sciencedirect.com/science

11. www.thespinejournalonline.com/article/S1529-9430(01)00016-X/abstract

12. ACAtoday.org

Chapter 14

1. Palmer, D.D. *The Chiropractor.*

2. http://www.naturesystems.co.uk/NS04.pdf

3. Null, Gary et al. "Death by Medicine."

4. "Time to Act on Drug Safety." *JAMA* 279 (1998): 1571-1573.

5. Czarnota, Henry S. *The New Zealand Report.*

6. Lef.org

Chapter 15

1. Parker, Steve. *The Wright Brothers and Aviation.*

Chapter 16

1. Ford, Carin T. *Heroes of American History , John F. Kennedy: The 35th President (Heroes of American History).*

2. Birkner, Michael J. Dwight D. *Eisenhower: America's 34th President (Encyclopedia of Presidents.*

Made in United States
North Haven, CT
10 November 2026

22086760R00134